The Tales
of a
Suffolk GP

ANDREW YAGER

British Library Cataloguing in Publication Data
A catalogue record for this book is available from the British Library.

ISBN 978-1-915463-61-6

Cover design and typesetting by Angela Selfe
Cover photograph by Charles Greenhough

Printed in the UK

This collection of short stories started as a thank you to my family and then migrated into a brief commentary on primary care around the millennium, which proved to be a therapeutic experience. The stories are organised into approximate date order: from just before the start of the 1982 Falklands War to the Covid pandemic in 2020/21. Consent has been sought and identities changed where necessary.

CONTENTS

1

FLEDGLING FIRST STEPS

1981

A ragtag army of fellow medical students crammed into a small office on the fifth floor of the medical school endocrinology building; and I mean ragtag! An exclusive club, united in a common bond. Exam failure.

Our fate awaited us. Commanding the room was a large desk, behind which sat the brooding figure of Chalky O'Riordan, lead physician and head of endocrinology at the medical school. Chalky was so named due to his specialist interest in disorders of calcium metabolism, about which he was a world authority. Chalky was due to be our supervisor and mentor for the duration of the repeat examination. The optimists among us had hopes of one-on-one tutorials and revision sessions with the great man, with pastoral help given gladly along the way. The pessimists talked of a fearsome reputation with no prisoners taken – ever.

Chalky had a large, domed, balding head atop dark Irish eyes, and a scowl that could vaporise. Fixing each one of us in turn with his gaze, he growled, 'Right you lot. You are a disgrace. There are four reasons for why you are all in here today. You are either too stupid, too lazy, drink too much, or indulge in too much fornication!'

Symptomatic of my quirky sense of humour, I couldn't help but smile as imperceptibly one or two of our motley crew nodded at each insult. One, two, three, four, full house for Steve. The same for John. I was probably a high score but took umbrage at the first three, whilst the fourth involved quite a lot of effort, actually.

The tirade continued. 'I do not want to see any of you ever again. You will leave this room, sort yourselves out and never come back. Any questions?'

Stunned silence. If anyone was holding a pin, now was not the time to let it drop.

'Now get out, the lot of you.'

That was it. Supervision, mentoring, tutorials, educational needs assessments were certainly not on Chalky's revision menu that day. We trooped down the stairwell shell shocked, undoubtedly demoralised, and reflecting on our bleak futures. In hindsight, just as I would have responded better to the hairdryer treatment of Sir Alex Ferguson had I been a footballer (rather than the intellectual encouragement of Arsene Wenger, or the mind games of José Mourinho), it was Chalky's hairdryer treatment that I needed to hear as a medical student, as for the preceding year I had not applied myself assiduously enough. So, his diagnosis and treatment were correct, but the process was bruising and not to be forgotten in a hurry. Painful as it was, Chalky's rollicking pushed me, reluctantly, onto the first rung of the vocational career ladder up which I knew I had to climb. It was a necessary first step.

My second dose of 'career enlightenment' came not in a single burst but over a prolonged period of six months whilst working in my first hospital job in Ipswich, for general surgeon Mr Bernard Hand. Stories of Bernard's working habits abounded, as he was renowned for working relentlessly long hours and expecting a similar commitment from his juniors, in what was tantamount to a medical boot camp, with grown men reduced to tears. On arriving, my first working rota lasted for twelve days on the trot, with five nights on call thrown in for good measure. It was one hundred hours a week for starters, during which time I did not leave the hospital and was permanently at Bernard's beck and call. By the end of this first twelve-day stretch, I was exhausted, ready to scream, and looking forward to two days back in London with my friends. Just a ward round and tidying up and handing over to do, and that was it. Freedom, fresh air and fun, albeit tired fun. But Bernard had other ideas!

'How did you find the on call last night, boy?' asked Bernard in his own inimitable way.

'Fine, thank you, sir. One or two cases of abdominal pain that we found difficult to fathom out, but otherwise everything went as well as can be expected,' came the hesitant reply, before elaborating further on the cases in turn.

'What are you doing over the weekend?' Bernard barked.

'Going back to London.'

'Not much then?'

'No, not really, no.'

'Well, in that case, we cannot have you struggling to diagnose abdominal pain on this ward, boy. I want you to go to the library at lunchtime, take out Zachary Cope's *Early Diagnosis of the Acute Abdomen* and read it through thoroughly over the weekend. It will not take too long as it is only a couple of hundred pages. If you read it properly, digest and understand it, your diagnostic skills will improve markedly. I will assess how much you have taken on board on the Monday ward round. Got that?'

I was crestfallen as my weekend's relaxation disappeared down the plughole. Each of Bernard's two hundred pages was punctuated with a pained rejoinder to keep my big mouth shut next time, although I was to find out during the subsequent six months and into my career that this book was a life saver, so let me elaborate.

Several years later, during a Saturday afternoon on call, I was asked to visit a seventy-five-year-old man who had returned from holiday feeling out of sorts with mild abdominal pain and diarrhoea. When questioned further, he attributed his symptoms to a German sausage eaten whilst away. However, on examination, his temperature was normal but his pulse raised, blood pressure low and abdomen tender with some increased muscle tone. My tacit knowledge was prodding my anxiety into acknowledging that these symptoms and signs do not point to the German sausage as the cause, whilst my explicit Zachary Cope knowledge was trying to make sense of it all. Could he have intra-abdominal bleeding? This was not a time to pontificate. Action was needed, and I decided to admit him to hospital, where he was found to have an early dissecting aortic aneurysm, subsequently successfully repaired at Addenbrooke's Hospital. You see, I had learnt something from that painful weekend in London reading Zachary Cope!

This was one of many lessons learnt during an extremely arduous but ultimately rewarding hospital attachment in Ipswich, working for a legendary figure who cajoled, frustrated, inspired, frightened, amused and ultimately heaved me further up the vocational career ladder. Medicine at long last made sense to me now. Increasing my knowledge base in this pressure cooker of an environment allowed me to love the responsibility of looking after and caring for the patients on the ward.

In 2009, the European Working Directive was applied to junior doctors, resulting in the abolishment of the long working hours I had worked and the adoption of a shift system. An unintended consequence of this policy change was the removal of the old 'firm' system that I experienced under Bernard Hand, where we worked in a hierarchical unit with support and role models usually evident. In order to fulfil the strictures of the Working Directive, shifts were introduced, and juniors were required to work according to a rota rather than a team or firm. The intention was to improve junior doctors' working environment, and although popular in some quarters, the European Directive changes have made no difference to depression, burnout and fatigue in the junior doctor ranks. I had relished the supportive medical boot camp under Bernard's tutelage and feel that a shift system working on my own, with no role model or ongoing support, would have left me disillusioned and disheartened.

My final step up the vocational ladder came when I left the hospital environment and entered into general practice. Almost from day one, I felt comfortable and in the correct milieu. I had felt ward work distracting and had struggled to concentrate on the problem at hand and communicate effectively with a patient. I never felt on top of the situation on the ward, whereas holed up in a general practice consultation room or house visit on my own was a different kettle of fish. I was able to get under the bonnet of the patient holistically and hopefully address their medical, social and psychological problems. It was duck-to-water stuff for me and a total relief to find a medical arena that I enjoyed. Starting with a shove from Chalky and Bernard, the slightly disillusioned and diffident medical student had been replaced with an ardent fledgling GP. To this day, I still do not quite understand this slow change in mindset, this rite of passage as expressed by Sir William Osler, one of the founding professors of Johns Hopkins Medical School a century ago: 'The practice of medicine is an art, not a trade; a calling, not a business; a calling in which your heart will be exercised equally with your head.'

There is a coda to this tale, however, involving father and son, son and father in a personal symmetry for me. I am standing in one of the great halls of Yale University, talking to Dermot O'Riordan in 2015. Previously, we had both won places on a diploma course at Yale, and during that time surgeon Dermot and I had become good mates. He was telling me about growing up in London, as his father had been a consultant endocrinologist. The cognitive penny dropped, and I enquired hesitantly,

'Dermot, was your father Chalky O'Riordan at The Middlesex Hospital?'

'That's him. The very same. Why, did you meet him?'

Did I meet him? Did I meet him? I preceded to regale him with the story of my one and only encounter with his dad, causing Dermot to reply through his laughter,

'That sounds like him. If it makes you feel any better, try being his son!'

I am at a medical meeting in Norfolk in 2000 talking to local GP Christopher Hand, Bernard's son.

'Your dad really turned my life around when I was his house officer, Christopher. I was so sorry when I heard that he had passed away. He was just the best.' With that, Christopher got out his wallet and unfolded a crumpled piece of paper with a *British Medical Journal* obituary of his father printed on it. He passed it hesitantly over to me, uttering, '*Mors vincit omnia*' – death conquers all.

'You are right . . . he was the best. Read this.'

The thing was, I didn't need to, as I also had a copy of the very same obituary in my own wallet.

2

KNIFE EDGE

1986

It is a cold Saturday morning in winter. The clock is ticking, and Annie (nickname Pom) and I are sleeping. The alarm rings, and a lazy hand presses the stop button. It is warm in bed, cold outside, and there is time for another five minutes' slumber. We doze on for another five, and then another ten. In our somnolent state, we are wrestling with the fact that on this morning, in just over an hour, we have an important interview. A really very important interview. On the other hand, we know it is cold outside, and it is cosy under the duvet. Thoughts traverse our minds, realising that we are getting mighty close to the point of no return and missing the interview deadline altogether. In the nick of time, concerns about letting our interviewers down stir us into action. The only problem is that we are on the Norfolk coast, and the interview is in Suffolk. We need to be out of the house and in the car in five minutes. It is not too late, and we can do this. Action! The foolhardiness and optimism of youth encapsulated in a Saturday morning lie-in.

Not that we had not prepared for this interview. It is just that a lie-in got the better of us, on this day of all days. Before I go back to this caper, some background is needed here. Annie and I had just finished our respective training schemes and tentatively accepted work in Rotorua, New Zealand. With slight misgivings about leaving our families, we had decided to see the world and work abroad for a year or two. Then, out of the blue, a general practice partnership opportunity in a highly respected health centre in Suffolk was presented.

'I know you are wanting to see the world, Andrew, but jobs like this come up once in a blue moon,' intimated Ian, my GP trainer, mentor and guru.

'I don't stand a chance, Ian. There are tens of applicants for this job at least.'

'I am telling you, give it a go. New Zealand can wait. General practice is so competitive these days. You may not get another chance.'

These were Ian's final words on the matter, and so give it a go I did. A scripted and informative curriculum vitae with references was posted off with due care and attention. Before we knew it, Annie and I had been invited to an interview in a few weeks' time, on what was to be the cold and frosty Saturday mentioned.

I know it was wintery weather, but how could we have even considered derailing such careful preparation for a job application with a lie-in? Benjamin Disraeli was quoted as saying that youth is a blunder, manhood a struggle; well this was a blunder of epic proportions and becoming more of a struggle by the minute. Anyway, Annie and I were up and off in our little Talbot Samba.

Tie, jacket, hair, tights, shaving, makeup were all dealt with in the car between King's Lynn and Thetford in a welter of conversation, clothing, exclamation, hot air, cold air and profanities. Ironically, we would not have made it nowadays, as the traffic is so much heavier, but make it we did, and bundling into the health centre, we were welcomed by one of the partners.

'Hello, Andrew and Annie. My name is Rob, and I am one of the partners here. Come on through.'

Rob was a young, windswept, bearded chap with a quiet, kind manner, dressed in jumper and jeans; he was more akin to a shepherd than the archetypal GP. I was cool with a shepherd as a partner but wondered whether I had needed to wear the tie, which had resisted my attentions whilst careering around the accident-prone King's Lynn roundabout on two wheels. I glanced across at Annie chatting to Rob; she looked a million dollars and up for the interview. In those days, general practice was a family affair, so, where possible, the partner of the applicant was also invited. Annie was enjoying this, and thank goodness she was by my side, as with her Irish lilt and charm, we were off to a flying start. Feeling half human myself now, my spirits soared as we progressed through to meet Dr Bill, the senior partner.

Bill was a well-spoken, kindly gentleman in his mid-fifties, dressed in sports jacket and tie and armed with pen and paper and a host of searching questions.

Bill and Rob, Rob and Bill extensively interviewed us. The proceedings started off with questions, with no stone left unturned, and then progressed to a relaxed conversation; finally, it turned into what felt like a bonding experience. Returning to our car, I exclaimed to Annie, 'I really like those guys.'

'So do I. They were both really caring chaps.'

'Do you know, I have a good feeling about this. I think we are going to get this job.'

How right I was, as following a second round of interviews, and the same relaxed, caring atmosphere, we did end up being offered the job at Botesdale Health Centre. Within the period of a few weeks, our life trajectory had changed; we now had to quickly decide between a journey into the unknown in New Zealand, or a journey into the equally unfamiliar in Suffolk. Annie and I have made three big decisions in our lives: deciding to marry, join Botesdale, and have children, all made on an intuitive and emotional level, augmented here and there with the occasional word of advice from friends and family:

'When choosing a partnership, Andrew, it is the other partners that matter, not the area or the building.'

'If you can see yourself fitting into the partnership then everything else will come out in the wash.'

'Do you think you will miss your families if you move to New Zealand?'

'You would be bonkers not to take up the Botesdale job, my son.'

How correct these words were, as Botesdale Health Centre and the area of North Suffolk have been inordinately kind to us. Annie and I sometimes reflect on that particular Saturday morning, however, and the likelihood of a slightly longer lie-in leading to a completely different outcome in our lives. It had been a decisive moment for us both, ignorantly perched on a knife edge, our futures in the balance. We were very fortunate to slither down the correct face of the blade that day.

3

'I NEED YOU HERE NOW, BOY'

1987

I remember a wise old sage of a GP asking me once, 'What is the most important item of equipment for an on-call GP, Andrew?'

'A medical bag?'

'Nope. Jump leads, son! Jump leads. You are so busy that you will leave your lights on and flatten your battery more times than you care to imagine. Without your car you're totally buggered!'

How right he was . . .

Twenty-four-hour responsibility before the 2004 GP contract really did mean responsibility for patient care round the clock, undertaken either as an individual practice or as a group, in a so-called GP co-operative. In the course of one generation, however, I have gone from being contacted by radio pager, stopping the car and phoning Annie from a telephone box, through to a commercial out-of-hours service with switchboard and a fully equipped fleet of cars. The old system had a certain charm but involved working long hours and feeling isolated and at times very vulnerable, with little support apart from the person answering the call at home, my rock Annie. There was some peripheral help from the 999 services, the local hospitals and social services on occasions, but the population thirty years ago viewed the GP as the first port of call. I found that as well as dealing with complex medical problems when on call, non-medical problems could arise that would completely derail what had been a relatively ordered day. These were the real rocks in the water when working alone at all hours – sometimes of my own making, and sometimes involving my car, without which, as you have already heard, I was totally buggered.

It was two o'clock in the morning on the cold, dark, dank edge of the fen on the Norfolk-Suffolk border where we lived. The telephone rang next to our bed, triggering the usual palpitations.

'Come quickly, Doctor. I'm in a hell of lot of pain,' Lennie gasped.

'Whereabouts is the pain?'

'My belly.'

'I will be along as quickly as I can.'

'I need you here now, boy!'

'Where do you live?'

'Church Hill.'

And that was it! Click! The call was high on desperation and low on detail. All was not lost, however, as I knew Lennie well enough to have an inkling of where he lived . . . or so I hoped!

Lennie was in agony, and without further ado, I jumped up and ran round the bedroom, looking for my clothes.

This was not a time for delay. Annie managed to achieve some semblance of sleep despite the bedside light, the rummaging and the general commotion. In a flash, I was out of the back the door and round to the grass drive where our sturdy white Ford Fiesta sat in the gloom. Car keys? They were not in my trouser pockets as usual, or in my jacket pockets. I thundered back upstairs, with Annie now realising things were amiss.

'What's wrong?'

'I have lost the car keys and got an emergency.'

With that, Annie was up and on the hunt too. Upstairs in the bedroom, and then downstairs to the kitchen. Back and forth, back and forth. Eventually, I went to look at the car again, where to my horror I saw the keys in the ignition with the car locked, having used the old trick of lifting the drivers handle whilst shutting the locked car door. Shit! Running back in, I declared, 'Where is the spare set, Pom?'

'Are they hanging up on the hook?'

'No!'

Oh my God. 'I need you here now, boy,' was resonating around my brain. High on desperation, low on detail! More rummaging, with the gnawing realisation that because of Lennie's manifest pain there was only one thing for it! I did not have time to do the old trick with a coat hanger or packaging tape, which I was accustomed to. You see, I had previous form with this sort of caper. Five years previously, whilst windsurfing on the River Orwell, I had been caught in my wetsuit with my car on the beach, tide coming in, and my keys locked in the car. On this occasion, a police officer miraculously appeared from nowhere with packaging tape coiled around the rim of his cap and rescued me, my dignity and my car! However, that was then, and this was now, with no such appearance likely at two o'clock in the morning on the edge of the fen.

So, before I knew it, there was a brick in my hand which then took itself through the passenger rear window. Smash! I was in. With the car started, I hurtled through the fen to Lennie's farmhouse on Church Hill. Boy, was I relieved to be on my way, despite the cold air on my neck and the crunch of glass in the footwell as I operated the pedals.

'I need you here now, boy!' OK, I am on my way now, I reassured myself.

Fortunately, my memory of Lennie's farm was correct, and despite some initial hesitation, I found the track down to his house, where a single 100W bulb above the porch shone forth through the mist. In through the back door and straight into the kitchen, I saw Lennie reclining almost supine in his armchair by the Aga.

'Where the hell have you been? You only live on the other side of the fen!'

A muted tone to the voice did not conceal the blazing, angry eyes and curl to the lip.

'It's a long story Lennie,' I replied before getting on to a more diagnostic footing, which included some basic questions and an examination. This was not a time for excuses.

It was evident that Lennie had an acute abdomen and was eventually diagnosed as having acute pancreatitis, one of the most painful conditions known to man. Analgesia was given and an ambulance called, with me sitting nearby until he was eventually taken to hospital. Few words were subsequently spoken, but the general air of dissatisfaction with my service hung in the air between us. The delay in my response time was probably only 15 minutes, but it felt like a long time to me, and an eternity to Lennie.

Needing the Fiesta for work meant that I took some time to get my window replaced, with a sheet of polythene making a dashing if noisy and cold replacement. For some reason, my car was never a symbol of suave medical sophistication. The high-end BMW or Merck were never on the menu for me. A grubby, white Ford Fiesta with polythene windows took some beating, however.

Following Lennie's discharge, I was keen to visit him, knowing that he had been unhappy, and with guilt still coursing through my veins, I ventured round to his farmhouse on the edge of the fen.

'Hello, Doctor, sorry I was sharp with you the other night,' Len stated with a wry smile and slightly clipped tones.

I grinned sheepishly and declared that he should look out of the kitchen window and see my repair work. After a brief explanation, the penny dropped, and from that moment on, we were firm friends. Lennie was bluff, robust and knowledgeable but a firm man of the country, who was undoubtedly better to have on side than otherwise. From time to time, I would subsequently see him in the surgery, and over the years we would share this tale. He understood that problems can happen in a working day and saw the humorous side to the problem of an urgent visit that night: a car incapacitated by trapped car keys, a brick and a smashed window!

Have I finally learnt my lesson, however? Well, I do keep jump leads ready to hand, but I also know exactly where the spare keys reside in our house at any given time!

4

LOTTIE

1989

The afternoon sun courses through the trees as I plod along the winding footpath through Rickinghall churchyard, on my way home from a dog walk. A notion takes root, and I veer off the path to a small headstone tucked away amidst a line of larger memorials. Lottie.

Reflecting on the events of over thirty years ago, and although sadness coils around my heart, my prevailing thought is one of hope. This story of parental strength and resilience needs airing.

CHERISHED MEMORIES OF
CHARLOTTE EMILY BAREHAM

15th June 1989 – 13th December 1989

Forever Loved
Forever Missed
Forever Ours

Lottie was the firstborn child of Richard and Nina, a vibrant, charming and attractive couple in their twenties. Recent residents of Suffolk, they had moved to the area with their parents and in a joint family venture taken over the management of a local pub. To the delight of the family, Lottie arrived on the scene relatively quickly. All was well until Lottie developed a blister the size of a 10p bit hours after birth, followed quickly by more blistering on different sites of her small body. A dermatologist was called and a skin biopsy undertaken, which revealed the characteristic picture of Severe Junctional Epidermolysis Bullosa. This is a very rare condition, characterised by severe blistering of skin, mouth and oesophagus, with only a handful of babies making it through to infancy. Unbeknown to themselves, Richard and Nina were genetic carriers of this condition, resulting in each of their children having a 1 in 4 chance of inheriting the fully blown defective skin, incompatible with life. With skin as fragile as the wings of a butterfly, the surface layers of skin and mucous membranes tear and separate at the slightest touch. These children are known as 'the butterfly children' as a result of this. Sadly, Lottie had inherited the most severe form of epidermolysis bullosa, rendering her short life to the palliative care equivalent of a burns victim, with no treatment or cure in sight.

Skin is a remarkable organ, the interface between our internal and external worlds; a water-resistant barrier protecting us from infection, and involved in heat regulation, sensation, absorption and excretion. We spend billions of pounds on the psycho-social elements of this organ while being largely indifferent to many aspects of its function. All things considered, skin performs remarkably well for the majority of us, considering the battering it gets, and it only breaks down with fatal consequences very rarely. Severe epidermolysis is one of those occasions, due to a genetic deficiency in the manufacture of the collagen strands that bind the superficial layers of the skin together, leading to catastrophic skin fragility.

After a relatively short stay in hospital, Richard and Nina returned home with Lottie swathed in gauze bandages and a soft protective head bonnet. This was my introduction to the most beautiful baby, remarkable for her radiant pale blue eyes and calmness. Nina and Richard had been instructed in hospital on how to undertake dressings, with feeding and nappy changes made all the more challenging by the fragile butterfly skin and membranes. Boy, did they rise to the challenge! Positive, energetic and purposeful in their love for Lottie, they met the daily problems full on, aided and abetted by Jo and Jane, our hardworking and caring district nurse and health visitor. None of us had looked after a baby with such a condition before, and whilst our inexperience was evident, we were prepared to learn, and learn quickly. Initially, Richard, Nina and Lottie would attend hospital; however, these trips gradually diminished as it became evident that there was no substantive treatment available. Gradually, we fell into a working pattern, with Nina and Richard in charge, making the major decisions. We were the ship's crew, with Nina the purposeful, clear-thinking, positive captain charting Lottie's course in this ill-defined and indeterminate journey, whilst Richard somehow managed to hold down a full-time job during this time.

Gradually, over the following six months, the ravages of the condition on little Lottie took their toll. Pain, anaemia, feeding difficulties, infection and fluid depletion all reared their ugly heads. Nina and Richard were losing the battle, but they never complained or wavered in their love and care for Lottie. On entering the house, there was always a calm and purposeful atmosphere, with Nina and Richard at the helm, confronting difficult decisions around analgesia, nutrition and fluid control on a daily basis. Eventually, however, enough became enough for poor Lottie, and she died peacefully in her parents' arms early in the morning of the 13th December. Having been part of the furniture for the last few weeks, I had asked Richard and Nina to ring me if things deteriorated, and so in the early hours I was asked to attend. On entering the room, there was Lottie lying in her cot, surrounded by her parents and grandparents, Mike and Pam, in peace at last. I ended up staying for a couple of hours, as there were quite a lot of formal issues to discuss initially, and it seemed inappropriate to rush off to the comfort of my bed at such a harrowing moment for those left behind. What did the five of us end up talking about at this distressing time? Our favourite Beatles songs; I suppose in an attempt to temporarily normalise and soften the harsh world this family were existing in.

Now, I did say at the beginning that this was a story of remarkable resilience, well unfortunately this couple were to be tested a second time, with further tragedy waiting around the corner. In an effort to make sense of and reverse the terminal nature of Lottie's life, Nina had fallen pregnant again during this time. At the time, this was one positive way of coping with Lottie's illness. The only problem was the 1 in 4 odds remained for this second pregnancy, with Nina and Richard deciding to travel down to King's College in London for a foetal skin biopsy to rule out a further case of severe epidermolysis bullosa. Late one afternoon, the result was phoned through by the clinic. 'Sorry, Nina, the result is positive. You now need to decide whether to proceed with the pregnancy or not.'

The word devastation does not do justice to the situation Nina and Richard were in now. This was their darkest hour, with life at its cruellest. They decided to terminate the pregnancy and take stock of the last year. They grieved but somehow managed to stay positive and strong, with a firm conviction that they would journey out of this personal nightmare. Many couples fall apart when tragedy strikes, but not Richard and Nina, who actually drew together and became closer in their relationship. If they could survive the last few months, they could get through anything. The metaphorical bar of tragedy was set so high now in their case that nothing life threw at them in the future would ever be as bad. They could cope with anything and were an example of personal fortitude on a monumental scale.

One morning after nearly a year, I saw Nina's name down on my surgery list. With slight trepidation, I ushered her into the room, where she quickly declared that she was pregnant again, and with a grim determination, she asked that we institute the same diagnostic tests as last time, with a trip to King's and a foetal skin biopsy. The only difference to her request this time was that the result would be phoned through to me in the surgery, and she asked if I would be prepared to come round after surgery at 6.30 to inform her of the good or bad news in person. I had been notified of the exact date of the result and asked my receptionist to put through any call from King's straight to me in my room. One late afternoon, a few weeks later, my desk phone rang. 'The nurse from King's College is on the line.'

'Thanks, Shirley, put her through.'

'Hi, this is the nurse from the foetal sampling unit at King's about a specimen taken from a patient of yours. She asked that you specifically take the call. I am really pleased to report that it is negative for epidermolysis bullosa!'

Eureka, they are in business! I was overjoyed, and after finishing my surgery in record time, I ventured round to their house. Now, that morning I had had a feeling in my bones that lightning would not strike three times and had put a bottle of champagne in my car as a celebratory token if called upon. This was to become the first and last time I delivered a laboratory test result brandishing a bottle of champagne. I knocked on the door and holding the bottle aloft declared 'Congratulations, the skin biopsy is normal. You are only allowed a small glass of this Nina, whilst the rest is for Richard and me!!'

So, the nightmare was over, with healthy baby Lydia born later in the year, followed quite quickly on her heels, after the same diagnostic test, by brother Henry. Born out of adversity, these two wonderful children have grown up into confident, successful adults; Lydia is married to Carl and has three small children of her own, Charlotte, Alice and Elizabeth. The family unit of eight all live within striking distance of each other and are extremely close, with the memories of Lottie never far from their thoughts. As stated on Lottie's epitaph, she is forever loved, missed and ours. Her memory and experience has fashioned the future and dynamic of this family to the degree that they will always be close, loving and in contact.

Now, I said at the start of this story that my abiding feeling whilst staring down at Lottie's headstone was one of hope, and why is this? Well, to encounter a couple so positive about their dealings with the world, believing that they will venture through the other side of any personal difficulties, gives me optimism for all of our futures. With significant global challenges on our doorstep, it is up to human ingenuity and spirit acting cohesively to resolve these problems. With people like Nina and Richard in the world, all will be well.

5

GWEN AND THE TORNADO

1989

I am strolling down the hill into Rickinghall with our two dogs, Albert and Paddy, when I see a familiar figure in the distance with grey bobbed hair, woollen coat, flat sensible shoes and a large wheeled shopping bag. Gwen takes a while to recognise me, making me question her vision; however, eventually her face lights up into the friendly warm smile which I had first encountered thirty years ago.

'What are you up to, Gwen?' I enquire, wondering about the destination of the huge shopping bag.

'I am on my way to Diss to fetch some shallots for planting,' she replies firmly and then chuckles in excitement.

Her twinkling eyes remind me of an adventure we went through together, and I can't resist asking.

'Do you remember the Tornado jet all those years ago, Gwen?'

'Ah yes, the airplane, I remember,' she replies quietly, with typical Suffolk understatement and then adopts a distant expression of thoughtful reminiscence. It had been an afternoon in December when Thor the god of thunder descended.

On that particular grey, cold and bleak afternoon, I had a visit scheduled to see Gwen's brother, Fred, who was convalescing at home following a prolonged period of time in hospital. Those were the days when we tried to visit patients on their return home from hospital to ensure all was progressing smoothly, check the medications and answer any remaining questions. With workload at its present level, this service has long become a thing of the past; however, on that afternoon, I was standing in the lounge talking to Fred when a roaring sound in the distance entered into my consciousness. I exchanged a glance with Gwen, whose face registered a quizzical smile. Quickly, the noise level intensified.

'Christ that's low!' I thought, realising the noise was a jet engine. I had thought this many times before in my life with the certain and reassuring knowledge that within a second or two the roaring sound would fade away and disappear. This time was different.

A crackling, tearing roar. Boom!

A deep bass rumble engulfed the timber-framed house, shaking what little foundations were present. The building swayed, plaster crumbled, and Gwen and I instinctively ducked our heads. The back door in the kitchen burst open with Cecil, Gwen's husband, staggering across the threshold and landing in a crumpled heap. I looked out of the open door and witnessed Armageddon coming to Suffolk. A stone's throw away in the back field was a crater, vaguely visible below a ball of flame and a huge mushroom cloud billowing into the sky.

Cecil was by now standing with a dazed and bemused expression on his face. 'Cor to heck! That was a jet . . . came over from Diss way and crashed itself in the meadow. Came too close for comfort as far as I can see.'

On proceeding to the back garden, there was not much to see apart from a black hole and smoke – lots of smoke. The acrid smell of aviation fuel was everywhere. Surviving this carnage did not look possible from where we were standing, when keen-eyed Cecil pointed up to the sky and shouted,

'Look. There are the pilots coming down with parachutes.'

Sure enough, along the flight path of the jet were two small figures with billowing white canopies, serenely floating earthwards.

Before engaging my brain, I shouted, 'Come on, Cecil, let's get after them and check they make it down alright.'

Why I said this, I don't know, but say it I did. I have heard stories of pilots ejecting and injuring or killing themselves, and something in me thought I could help. At no stage did I consider that help was a relative term and that helping armed with a bag containing only a stethoscope and some antibiotics could be problematic. It was probably, on closer consideration, a bridge too far for Cecil too. Leaving Gwen and Fred to deal with the aftermath of an explosion in their back garden, Cecil and I jumped into my white Fiesta and set off on a madcap caper through and over the fields to try and follow the descent of the two pilots. We were all action, fuelled by adrenaline, with little rational thought on my part. With relative ease, we could see the shock of the white parachute material against the brown corduroy of a nearby ploughed field. On subsequent reflection, the distance between the pilot's descent and the crash site was close enough to indicate that they had ejected at the last second to avoid the jet careering into the village where I had very much been present. Brave chaps, we found one pilot lying on the soft soil holding his ankle and looking up at me with an anguished expression.

'I have just written off 12 million quid, 12 million quid.' He continued repeating this mantra through clenched teeth while holding his leg. As if from nowhere, his co-pilot, who appeared of senior rank, calmly ambled over and reassuringly chipped in through the 12 million quid refrain, 'Don't worry bud, it can't be helped, and we brought the bird down in a field, so no harm done. There was nothing else for it.' This relaxed and calm mien was impressive stuff given the circumstances! Whilst waiting for the ambulance, I checked the ankle – a probable fracture – and then we proceeded to keep the pilot warm and offer analgesia and comforting words regarding the lost 12 million pounds. No doubt there were other witnesses who had put two and two together, as the ambulance was quickly on the scene. We helped load the pilot onto the ambulance, and having a surgery to hurry back to, and journalists to avoid, Cecil and I took our leave.

Returning to the cottage, we found Fred and Gwen engrossed in conversation and pointing to the crater: a black, smoking void startlingly close to their house. Fred's hospital discharge was by now placed on the back burner by us all, as there were more pressing matters to discuss, such as how lucky we all were to be alive! Thinking about it, I am not sure we ever got round to dealing with Fred's discharge properly, if at all!

We now have the luxury of the internet, and looking up this incident I was interested to find the Aviation Safety Report of the incident on Wikibase. It details the crash as being due to aileron failure, with the jet damaged beyond repair and subsequently written off. Now, I have seen a car written off by an insurance company when repair on another day and in another age would have been possible; however, the understated 'damaged beyond repair' in this Aviation Safety Report raised a smile. When the four of us looked into that smoking chasm, at the bottom of Gwen's garden, filled with the odd, black, charred, twisted aluminium fragments, there was nothing discernible left to recognise, let alone repair. This was some write off.

Back to the present, and Gwen's distant expression was now replaced by her familiar kind smile.

'We were lucky that plane missed the house, Doctor.'

'Yes, we were lucky, Gwen, very lucky indeed,' I agreed, thinking that another fraction of a degree in aim and an earlier ejection by the courageous pilots might have resulted in a very different outcome for my home visit on that grey afternoon in winter. I suppose being killed by a fighter jet whilst on a GP home visit was covered by my life insurance policy!

Wishing Gwen well on her trip to Diss, our thoughts shift from the Tornado jet to shopping for shallots in the blink of an eye. Such is life. In the blink of an eye, everything can change.

6

IMAGE PROFESSIONNELLE

1990

For many years, now, there has been a GP delegation involved with Compiegne via the Bury St Edmunds Twinning Association. This particular year, Annie and I were invited along to fly the flag for Blighty and pair up with a charming French GP and his wife, Jean-Luc and Mariange. An enticing long weekend of easy travel by coach and ferry with the committee, followed by mayoral receptions, garden parties and a picturesque early morning trip to Paris awaited us. The perfect juxtaposition of suave Englishness meeting Gallic flair. What could possibly go wrong?

Vomiting in a coach loo is nigh on impossible, that's a fact. I discovered this on our return to Calais, journeying home. At over six feet tall, crouching to chunder is a no-no; having no option, I adopted the jack-knife position. Splatter, audible groan, and more splatter. My grey flannels and shoes are a write off. Return to seat with pale, embarrassed face, a shuffling passage along the rows of seats. Wrinkled noses and sympathetic smiles from the blazers and twin sets within the delegation.

Oh no, more torture from the coach driver.

'Right everyone, we are at the ferry now, and I am closing the coach. The restaurant is open for refreshment, so make your way across the car park. Please return in two hours.'

'Pom, I can't go into a restaurant vomiting like this. I need to lie down.'

It was then that I saw a goods train, doors open, about 100 metres away.

'Pom, you go to the restaurant with the others, and I am going to find a place to lie down on that goods train!'

Desperation facilitates ever more extreme action. Climbing up into the carriage and onto some straw, I was able to lie down. Relief and some sleep. Groan! Vomit and groan, mindful that if I felt a clunk, I needed to hop off this goods van as soon as. A trip to Bordeaux was not on the twinning agenda!

Boarding the ferry, there was more olfactory aversion from the twinning team, but this was now accompanied by the not so hidden rictus of disgust at the matted straw and vomit caking my jacket.

'Pom, I am sorry, but I can't sit in a ferry lounge vomiting like this. I am going to sit outside, despite the weather. You stay inside with the others.'

I sat on the slatted outdoor bench for the duration; the cool, damp breeze soothing my fever. I must have been a helpless, sorry sight.

We arrived home at last. The previously semi-suave English GP exiting the coach on Angel Hill, Bury

St Edmunds, at the end of the twinning visit, had undergone a metamorphosis; the neat jacket and flannels replaced by damp hair and dishevelled clothes caked in vomit and straw. How easy it is to be rendered incapacitated by infection within hours, our human vanities rendered meaningless. As the other members of the party climbed into their BMWs and Jaguars, we started up our trusty white Ford Fiesta. Oh dear, one final indignity as we watched everyone scoot off; a flat battery compounded the misery!

I remembered the wise old owl: 'Jump leads, son. Jump leads.'

So with the collapse of my professional image on this particular French exchange trip, I got to thinking about the evolution of the medical dress code during my career.

My own dress has varied over the years from white coat initially in hospital, through to jacket and tie, to no tie, no long sleeves, and finally to theatre scrubs. Image has played its part in this transition, but infection control appears to have held sway over the major changes, with white coats jettisoned in 2007 in the UK due to infection risk and cost of daily laundry, and ties and jewellery due to MRSA. Scrubs were necessary with Covid in 2020, so it was full circle from clinical uniformity to individual choice and back again in forty years. When I had had a choice over clothing, personal comfort and relaying a relaxed competency to the patient were important, albeit backed up by warmth, a multitude of pockets to carry stuff in and a slight scruffy edge.

For the profession as a whole, the uniformity of today's theatre scrubs and the white coat of yesteryear alleviate the vagaries of individual dress, which always risked resulting in cultural, religious and demographic clashes within the workforce. Even a glance back just ten years brings to mind dress codes from different medical schools that resulted in a cultural dispute.

To quote photographer Bill Cunningham, however, 'Fashion is the armour to survive everyday life.' Doctors are not alone in needing to express their personality and culture through dress, but with a tide of blue, green and red scrubs currently engulfing the NHS in the middle of the pandemic, is the die cast for evermore? With health managers now booted and suited, is dress code a metaphor for the uniformed clinical worker bee and managerial drone bee power play within the NHS? I am sure there will be further evolution of the dress code, as I cannot think of many professional groups who have seen as much change as the medics over the last fifty years. The question is, will the clinicians assert a future dress code autonomy, or will there be further large-scale shifts relating to infection control, the patient-facing nature of the job, and possibly managerial coercion. Space suits next?

7

BRIDGE HOUSE

1991

Annie had spent an afternoon having tea under the apple tree in Bridge House garden with Jeannie, a firm friend and fifty years her senior. One particular conversation had been of interest, which was that Jeannie was thinking of selling Bridge House and wondered if we would be interested in buying it.

It was a fact that when on call the whole family was housebound, as Annie had to be at home to answer the telephone when I was out. On call came around every third day and night in those days, making for a significant slice of our lives spent around the house and in the garden. If a third of our family life was to be tied to the home, then it made sense to make that home as pleasant as possible. And so the offer from Jeannie was to change our lives. Situated on the periphery of the health centre village, Bridge House was a nicely sized and beautiful timber-framed Suffolk hall house surrounded by a large garden.

We didn't countenance saying no to the offer, and moved swiftly on to the conveyancing formalities, conducted with impeccable politeness by Bill and Jeannie. Bill, an ex-colonel in the Norfolk Regiment

(9th foot), and first off his landing craft on D-Day, phoned the surgery asking me to return his call at my leisure.

'I have got one or two things to discuss about the sale, Andrew. As the sun is now over the yardarm, do you fancy coming round for a chat and toddy after surgery?'

On arrival, a stiff whiskey was pressed into my hand with Bill declaring,

'I was pinned down by a sniper in Normandy for two days and surrounded by bandits in Korea for two weeks, but nothing compares to the stress of moving house, Andrew!'

With a great deal of kindness, patience and the odd toddy from Bill and Jeannie, Annie and I found ourselves moving into Bridge House.

Our first action on moving in was to install an external BT bell that allowed us to hear the telephone ring from the garden, therefore allowing us to spend time outside when on call!

We are still there some thirty years later, and with our family flying the nest, our heads tell us that we need to move into a warmer, smaller, more modern and easier to maintain property. The problem is that this old place has seeped into our souls, and our hearts cannot make the break, with the memories of our family, friends and youth, the smells, the creaks, the idiosyncrasies, and the perception that this old place has a personality of its own. There are the Christmases when my family came to stay and the Easters when Annie's parents visited; coming home with our new born babies in our arms, the sweet children's parties, the not so sweet teenage parties, the fun, the games, the banter, and the squabbles of a family doing its best. All within these lath and plaster walls.

I have been asked in the past what it is like to live and work in the same village, and whether we have had a constant stream of people knocking on our door. With the time now to deliberate this question, my reply has several strands. Our village neighbours have always been incredibly polite and respectful of our situation. I have always looked at the role of the local GP as not being any different to the role of, for instance, the electrician, plumber or policeman living in the village, contributing to the social fabric of the community and at times needed in a dire emergency. The very odd call is part and parcel of this social contract and commitment, with stories of knocks on the door having entered into the family lore of living in Bridge House.

So, we have had Herman coming round with a goose at Christmas, followed by Lindsay with a duck from his mum Dulcie. Joey walking down to ours on Christmas day under the misapprehension that we could provide the final answer to a crossword puzzle, and after wrestling with the problem for a millisecond happily settling for a sherry. An agitated motorcyclist dancing on the doorstep, excitedly pointing to his helmet where a bee was lodged in his ear canal, extricated with tweezers and a sigh of relief. A chap with a rifle and an angry look on his face hoping to shoot the dog who attacked his own dog . . . I viewed this handful of calls as part and parcel of village life and too infrequent to get upset about, although, hang on, maybe I did get upset by the chap with the rifle.

Thinking about it, we have had more kind neighbours rocking up at all hours on our doorstep returning our errant Cocker spaniel than patients requesting medical help! I was also aware of a sense of accountability and lack of anonymity if living in the practice locality, in that being part of the community you feel an ill-defined pressure to deliver high-performing services to the neighbourhood on a daily basis. This may increase the pervasive stress around the job, but I think it can be a force for improvement and engenders a sense of belonging. As a partnership, we were always on the scout for ways to improve the services offered, driven by accountability and a desire for excellence. When out of hours responsibility was removed from GPs, we were concerned that this change would possibly have a negative impact on the community and took steps to deliver improved services in other ways, such as setting up an Xray and ultrasound service.

I found the lack of any commute a huge benefit of working and living locally, freeing up time, saving energy and allowing more contact with my family, no matter how fleeting. Sharing the early morning train to London from Diss with the regular commuters on several occasions has made me realise that any disadvantages of living and working in the same locality are eclipsed by all the advantages, such as being able to drop in to Bridge House on the way through from a visit to grab a snack and have a quick chat with Annie, or deal with some crisis. Our window cleaner of twenty years was mightily relieved when I showed up following a 999 call from daughter Hannah and his subsequent arrest for burglary!

So where are we now that Annie and I are weighing up the decision to move or not, stick or twist? It is this old house again exerting its presence. Bill and Jeannie also found that Bridge House had seeped into their souls. A few years ago, Kit, their son, phoned and asked whether we would be happy to host a tea for family and friends in Bridge House following an interment service for Jeannie's ashes in the church nearby. Having moved around the world in army service, Kit explained that his parents viewed Bridge House as their spiritual home. Annie and I were delighted to offer something in return for the conversation underneath the apple tree many years ago and reconnect with the family who had occupied this house a generation before ourselves. A shared dialogue, a common bond and a mutual love of Bridge House.

8

'TEACHING POINT'

1997

Botesdale Health Centre has been a training practice for young doctors wanting to enter a career in general practice for over fifty years. During this time, there has been a series of doctors within the practice who gave of their time training these new recruits, myself included. Over my working life at Botesdale, I was fortunate to have over 35 trainees under my wing, all adding interest, energy and a sense of scrutiny to the working day. As well as relating to the trainees on a medical footing, I found it important to understand them as people, so as to make the most of their educational opportunities. We had academics, comics, introverts, extroverts, the hardworking, not so hardworking, argumentative and easy-going through the door all needing education, a sense of vocation, and nurturing. Usually it was easy; occasionally it was like pulling teeth. Erik was one of the easy ones!

Twenty years ago, primary care in Holland was in the doldrums, and in a similar position to the UK now. Training practices were hard to come by for Dutch doctors, and so there was a steady stream of talented trainees migrating across The North Sea. Erik was such a doctor, leaving the Hook of Holland on a ferry to travel to Harwich accompanied by his lovely wife Simone, herself an accomplished lawyer. With excellent English, good interpersonal and medical skills, kindness, and an extremely dry sense of humour, which I believe is mandatory in Holland, Erik joined our ranks at the health centre. It wasn't just the humour that we all took pleasure in; it was the prelude to the delivery of the amusing comment that raised a smile. When about to offer up a witticism, Erik would pause, clear his throat with an 'Agghm,' and then deliver the punchline. Usually, a knockout punch too. Let me continue this story with an example.

It was Saturday and a bright spring morning in Norwich. We had just started the early morning shift at seven. A call came in from a mum saying that her eight-year-old epileptic daughter was having a prolonged seizure and could we come straight away. As part of my obtaining the address, I asked the make and colour of the car in the drive, as it can be easier to find a car than the number or name on a door. Erik, myself, and a relief driver were out of the on-call base and into the car like bats out of hell in view of the nature of the call. Trying to be a model of educational enlightenment on the way there, I offered up, slightly pompously, a teaching point to Erik: 'Always get the details of the car in the drive as it can save time.'

'OK,' he said, in a muffled, unimpressed tone from the back seat.

We then went on to discuss the management of status epilepticus, where a seizure lasts for more than 5 minutes. This was potentially serious, at times frightening to deal with, and so it was good to run through the guidelines, which slightly allayed the anxiety coursing through my veins.

Unfortunately, the relief driver was no Lewis Hamilton, and by the time we reached the house, I was like a coiled spring. Carrying one silver examination bag each, we flung the doors of the car open and ran up the drive to the house, where the car described on the call was parked. Knock, knock, the door opened, and there were two young girls standing in the doorway.

'Is mummy in?' I enquired, with an air of urgency in my voice.

'She's upstairs,' replied the older of the two girls.

Our arrival was straight out of the SAS training manual. We were in and up those stairs in a flash, primed to deal with the emergency. There we found a shocked man in his 40s desperately trying to cover his torso with a dressing gown, and struggling. With not a stitch on, and one sleeve inside out resisting his attempt at modesty, he exclaimed quite politely given the circumstances,

'Who the fucking hell are you?'

Where is the mum who made the call, I thought. I looked him in the eye, where I again saw written across his shocked face, 'who the hell are you?' The penny dropped. Oh No! My response was a masterly example of touchy-feely, doctor–patient communication.

'Sorry, wrong house! Come on Erik!' I turned around and careered down the stairs and out the front door, Erik hot on my heels. Bang.

No explanation, no apology, no communication, nothing.

Leaving this poor bloke to continue his Saturday morning lie-in, or not, we were off around the back of the house. Why the back, you may ask? Answer: your guess is as good as mine, and I have no idea to this day. More madness, as we trooped between the two semi-detached houses through their gardens and over their fences. It was then that I heard Erik behind me clear his throat, 'Ahhgm.'

Oh no, here we go, what is Erik going to say now, at my most embarrassing hour? Then delivered in a voice that sounded more rumination than vocalisation but just loud enough for me to hear,

'Some teaching point!'

'Not now, Erik,' as I stifled a laugh. Now was not the time for humour, as we tramped through and over the boundary on our way to the emergency.

We reached the correct door. Knock, knock, and there was a relaxed-looking mum standing in the doorway, 'Hello, Doctor, thanks for coming so quickly, she is fine now. The fit stopped of its own accord, and I have everything under control.'

'Coming quickly'? Our journey felt like it had taken an age. You have no idea, I thought, but then that's adrenaline for you. We entered calmly and checked the child over before giving the mum advice in case of further problems. Our final act was to ask the mum to apologise to her neighbour on our behalf for our rude and alarming intrusion. Relief, another call finished and on to the next one.

Some teaching point indeed, and never to be forgotten in the annals of Botesdale Health Centre teaching lore. On sharing this story with other GPs and nurses over the years, I have heard other hair-raising tales of mistaken addresses, ranging from the incorrect person admitted to hospital through to the incorrect person administered an enema! A lesson learnt indeed, and we all need to openly reflect on the errors of our ways. This is not easy in the current climate of name and shame, recently exacerbated by the Dr Bawa-Garba case, but necessary all the same to reduce individual errors and make our organisational systems safer. To create the sort of arena for open discussion and learning will take political courage of gargantuan proportions, but happen it must.

After that Saturday morning jaunt, I was more careful about parked cars in shared drives and diving into houses. A lesson learnt, and not really the intended teaching point!

9

A SUFFOLK STOIC

1997

When I first travelled on the London Liverpool Street train towards Ipswich, crossing the Manningtree mudflats straddling the Stour Estuary into Suffolk, I was spellbound. Since that day, I have been entranced by the beautiful countryside, and enchanted by the people of Suffolk. I was on the train for a job interview at the old Anglesea Road Hospital in Ipswich, and it was on subsequently taking up the job that I first heard of 'The Suffolk Stoic Syndrome.' This was a term of respect used by some of the surgical staff to describe a particular group of tough, non-complaining patients who would play down their problems and struggle on regardless. I was warned to not necessarily accept their symptoms at face value and delve more deeply into the problem, as the diagnosis could be a lot more serious than initially presented. Stan was such a person. A hardened man of the soil not prone to complaining or worrying.

Annie and I were very fortunate to become acquainted with Stan, as we ended up buying his cottage on the edge of a fen, straddling the Norfolk-Suffolk border near the source of the Little Ouse. One of the draws of the cottage was Stan's wonderful garden. During the sale negotiations, I realised that Stan was having second thoughts about moving, as he loved his garden, which he had tended for over fifty years. So, one day, I suggested that he consider returning to his old house whenever he wanted and help us with the garden on a paid basis. Stan's face lit up at the idea, with Annie and I gaining a skilled gardener during a very busy time in our lives. After four years, we subsequently moved to Bridge House, but the arrangement stuck, with Stan working on the garden and treating it as his own.

For the next ten years, Stan could be found dressed in jacket, tie and polished shoes, cigarette dangling from lower lip, working his magic. Within a few months, he had the garden in shape, and from then on it became a thing of beauty and wonder. The lawn was a uniform green with sharp edges, moss free and not a mole in sight. The bushes and shrubs were each tightly shaped, with the vegetable garden bursting with produce. Apart from the trusty old Hayter Harrier mower, everything was done by hand, using sharpened tools and muscle. He would come in and sit in our kitchen for coffee mid-morning, disappear for a liquid lunch and return home late afternoon. Always quiet, calm and dignified, he had a dry wit enhanced by a throaty chuckle and cough. With our young, growing family, he became a source of help and constancy for Annie and me.

Then one day Stan informed us that he had developed some worrying symptoms and asked what he should do about it. He continued gardening with a spring in his step, a smile and a cheerful wave. Despite hospital treatment, his condition worsened, but did he miss a day? No. Did he complain? No. He followed his usual routine, with little talk of his condition, as from his point of view there was no point. He had sought treatment, which had not helped, and there was nothing for it but to soldier on living his normal outdoor life, taking each day as it comes, especially if the sun was shining and the wind blowing. Gradually, he became frailer and paler but still did the work of ten men, altering his routine not one jot. He began to struggle, really struggle, but he still didn't waiver in his fortitude. Annie and I watched from the sidelines as his life force slowly diminished and retracted, helping where we could. He took a few pain killers offered, but that was it.

At the beginning of his final week, he arrived looking dreadful, and with spade and shears in hand, he carried on doing some light work quietly. He left early that day, without having had a pint at lunchtime, and never returned. The next day his wife Sybil rang saying that Stan had taken to his bed and could he have something for the pain, which by now had become unbearable. I visited him, and with the help of the district nurses we were able to help; however, the pain returned in the night. He wouldn't let Sybil call me. Why? Because he knew Annie was days from delivering our daughter and did not want to disturb her. He tolerated the unbearable for us, our family. The following day, infused with guilt, admiration, and affection, I was able to help his discomfort, and that night he died peacefully, three days after laying down his tools for the final time. Hannah was born the following day; a joyous reminder of the circle of life, which Stan himself would have quietly understood.

Now, I am no gardener, but much of what I know about gardening came from Stan. I often hear his voice in the garden when needing advice. However, what I really learnt from him, though, was how to live a dignified, joyful and steadfast life through adversity and the final test which we all face. Stan made it look easy, and I know it's not. With sadness in my heart, I am very proud to count this 'Suffolk Stoic' as a friend.

10

HANDBRAKE TURNS

CIRCA 1998

If you were to ask me what my relationship with my car is, I would reply that I am an A to B man, with a desire for function over style. People in the know will assert that this is just as well. At one stage, I had a tough little pillar-box red VW Polo, which, whilst not my pride and joy, was a source of affection in view of its reliability. In all weather conditions, it was always ready for the off and never let me down; however, on one occasion it did go walkabout.

In days gone by, our visiting lists were monumental, with up to 20 visits or more sometimes recorded. It was vital to get a shift on, compute the geographical order of the visits before setting off to minimise the distance and have a snack at the ready at all times. During one particularly busy winter, I remember Rob had a catering pack of Mars bars on his back seat! Alright, alright, I have got my excuses in, and now for the story, but suffice it to say that I was up to my eyeballs in visits.

On this particular day, my first visit on the list was two young children who had been coughing all night and were now in bed with fevers. Not wanting to delay, I was off like Sterling Moss, and parked on the hill by the side door of the house. They were ill with chest infections, but not seriously so, and I spent some time giving treatment instructions to mum along with advice on when to call again if they did not improve or deteriorated. All pretty straightforward stuff and on to the next visit, until I opened the door of the house and looked for my car, which had vanished.

'Shit, some bastard has stolen my car. Not now, not today,' I shouted to myself.

Whilst reflecting on the rocketing crime statistics in Suffolk, I happened to look down the hill.

'Oh my God.'

Down the hill, across the main road, up the bank and into the hedge was my red Polo.

'You daft plonker. You left the handbrake off!'

Now the hard part. Running down the hill, I worried that someone may have been injured and my car damaged. I tried to convey an image of nonchalance and the everyday while my alter ego was repeatedly screaming,

'Oh my God. Idiot.'

Arriving at the car, I could not discern a body under the chassis or any apparent damage; however, the car was backed up the bank at a forty-five-degree angle with the rear in the hedge. Just as I was climbing up the bank and thinking I might have got away with this calamity, further humiliation arrived in the form of an old Suffolk boy on his bicycle, known for his humour and love of village gossip.

'Morning, Doctor.'

'Morning,' I replied cheerfully with an all is well with the world tone in my voice and a pathetic self-conscious wave.

Then I heard a chortling sound coming from him as he rode away hot foot to inform all and sundry in the pub about what he had just witnessed . . . that silly old GP has really excelled himself this time!

The same thing happened to new partner in the surgery Dr Tim. Coming to the end of a long on-call shift at tea time is not normally the ideal way to celebrate your wedding anniversary. That is what Tim faced that evening and on phoning wife Anna took the practical, but not necessarily the most romantic, route to mark the occasion.

'Hello, Anna, I have finished my shift. Fancy a kebab? I can drop by the Turkish takeaway in Diss on my way home if you like?'

Anna agreed to the offer, with at least one doner and one shish in the offing. Tim parked his mint green VW Passat Estate Coupe in the market square, and a famished Dr Cooke barrelled down the street to the venue well known for celebrating anniversaries! Fifteen minutes later, the old romantic strolls back up the hill and is presented with a slightly confused sight in the market square, where there is a mint green VW Passat Estate Coupe firmly lodged into the large window of Hopwood's, the local clothes outfitter. He regaled me with an account of the same quasi-nonchalant but panic-stricken walk that I remember so well towards the disaster scene; a wave and reassuring noises to the small crowd assembled around the car, all asking similar questions.

Who owns this car? Where has it come from? Who does this sort of thing? His anxiety of dealing with the onlookers was mitigated by the relief in seeing that the shop window was intact. By a minor miracle, the car had rolled down the marketplace hill and crunched into the solid wooden stanchion of the window, with the glass untouched. The rear bumper was a different kettle of fish, however, but with relief coursing through his veins and the smell of several kebabs in his nostrils, Tim quickly waved once more to the assembled folk and shot off to his anniversary. Mission accomplished.

Before I finish, let us briefly explore 'who does this sort of thing?'

Well, judging by the number of You Tube videos, handbrake misadventures are not uncommon; however, an honest answer to this question requires a little more explanation, as motoring mishaps appeared to happen quite regularly at Botesdale Health Centre.

Firstly, we were not too precious about our cars, always in a rush to get to home visits in far-flung rural areas involving farm tracks and muddy lanes, and our minds were on other matters. So maybe with time this led to a certain recklessness regarding the treatment of our vehicles. Not that I didn't value my chariot, which carried around a varied array of medical treatments, accessories and equipment at all hours with relentless reliability.

Nowadays, GPs spend more and more time in their medical premises, as this is a more efficient use of time. Why spend hours in a car as a rural GP every day when more patients can be seen in the same time by staying at base camp? This equation was determined when I retired from the partnership and the practice and decided to employ a paramedic, Andy, to undertake the majority of the visits. I thought this was an interesting and bold move. Once Andy got used to the cultural shift from moving from the front-line vans, as he called them, to primary care, he became an important adjunct to the practice team. Good communication skills, savvy, above average medical knowledge in emergency medicine and growing primary care clinical skills, he developed into the role of the primary care paramedic. We will see more and more people like Andy in health centres across the country, as the problems with training and recruitment of GPs continue unabated. Recently, I read a report of a practice in Leicester that audited their patient contacts and found that up to 33% of patients could have been seen by another health professional instead of a GP. This change is fine as long as the professionals who enter into this uncharted territory, such as pharmacists, physician associates, and paramedics, are managed closely, with governing body support extended from on high. From a personal point of view, much of the richness, colour and insight into how people live, which I loved, comes from home visits, and as such the GPs left behind in the practice will miss out on this. People like Andy are undoubtedly the beneficiaries of this workforce change, and as far as I am aware his car still remains in a reasonable condition, with no hair-raising stories of hills, handbrakes, or kebabs. Give it time, give it time!

11

THE LORD OF THE DANCE

1999

Dance, dance wherever you may be,
I am the Lord of the Dance, said he.

Staggering towards the beach in Cornwall, with all the paraphernalia an afternoon by the sea entails – windbreak, body boards, rucksack, and possibly even the kitchen sink – our family slowly migrates down the track from our holiday home. Not far to go now. Just up and over the considerable bank of dunes and we are there. Flip-flop, flip-flop. Hang on a moment, there is someone shouting above the wave noise and the metronomic slap of our flip-flops. It is sister-in-law Moira, wild-eyed and frenzied, with legs pumping through the soft sand dunes.

'Andrew, Andrew, a man has been stung by a wasp and is laid up in the coastguard's hut! Come on, run.'

Dropping my considerable cargo, I was off down the dunes, into the hut. I was greeted by two not so chilled Aussies, fear coursing across their tanned faces. Lying on a bench was a pale, clammy and incoherent fifty-year-old chap, with a fast, thready pulse. A wasp had apparently appeared from nowhere and stung the patient on the neck. Staggering along the beach, he then needed help getting to the coastguard's hut. The air ambulance had been called already for what appeared to be a case of anaphylactic shock. Acute anaphylaxis has always been one of my bête noires. It is a medical googly ball that can affect any of us, even the young and fit. The coastguard did not have access to adrenaline, so it was a question of basic support whilst we waited.

Then I heard it. The rhythmic thwump, thwump of a helicopter rotor blade in the distance. Airborne salvation as the poor chap clung on. Landing on the firm, wet sand, the crew ran into the hut armed with bags, bustle and competence. Finishing their assessment, they declared, 'It's acute anaphylaxis . . . we'll transfer him by air to hospital immediately for treatment.'

But that was a good 30 miles away, I thought, my mind racing . . . it was at least half an hour door to door. Looking at him now, he would not make it.

Before I knew it, I had piped up from my position in the corner. 'Hang on, he is in shock, and should he not have a shot of adrenaline first. He may not survive the journey.'

This is when things got interesting, as I half expected a retort of some kind, a comment along the lines of 'who the hell are you?' The reply, when it came, threw me off-kilter slightly. 'If you really think so. We are not allowed to give it, but we do have some. Here you are, if you want to give it a go?' Unzipping a pocket in his orange flying suit, the crewman brandished a preloaded syringe. I checked the dose and then injected it into the patient's thigh. No time for doubts to surface, no messing around, and no dissent from within the hut. We then proceeded to get the patient onto a stretcher and into the helicopter as quickly as possible. With colour and responsiveness improving, I saw a hint of a wave from the patient before the door shut, the rotors started, and off they went.

Leaving the assembled ring of onlookers, I trundled back to the family, perplexed and troubled, with several unexplained questions. Were the crew pilots or paramedics? Why did they carry adrenaline if they were not able to administer it? Why did they not ask who I was or what I did? Where was the ubiquitous paperwork on which the NHS feasts? By injecting the adrenaline, why did I rush headlong into a situation that could have resulted in potential professional harm? Remember that this was over twenty years ago and adrenaline autoinjectors were less prevalent than now. My curious sense of duty means that I have to jump in with both feet and get involved to the nth degree whatever the potential cost to me as a person or doctor. I am like an automaton, wound up, balls out with brain barely attached and ready repeatedly to do my dance. This was not the first time, nor would it be the last, and so I will illustrate with a different incident, different time – but oh dear, similar behavioural trait.

Night is falling and I am staggering blindly over rough terrain high in the Himalayas, hanging on to a yak.

I am descending from the settlement of Lobuche at an altitude of 16,000 feet, over a glacial moraine in the dark, valiantly transporting a Swedish chap encephalopathic with altitude sickness. What the fuck, I thought, you are at it again, dancing to the duties of a doctor tune again, without fully thinking things through. Night time without any equipment, sub-zero temperatures, a patient strapped to a yak, and no way of communicating with the yak herdsman. Exhausted after a day plodding around Everest Base Camp, here we go again, although it has to be said there were benefits to my own physical state from descent, as altitude sickness is just that: sickness. All the herdsman understood was that we were taking the patient down the mountain to the next village, paid for by money filched from the incapacitated Swede's wallet. You see, my plan followed the basic mantra at the time. 'There are three rules in treating altitude sickness: get the patient down, down, down.'

Simple, really, except not so simple on this occasion, as I did not know this plan would work, where we were going, and where we would rest up in the next stop. Pheriche? With the cold seeping in, why had I bought my Hollofil jacket and boots on the cheap in the January sale? Why hadn't I brought with me better equipment and more provisions? What was I doing going halfway up Everest on the back of a Blacks winter sale? All I had was what I was dressed in and some cash in my pocket! I suspect the bastard Swede perched on top of the yak was better equipped than I was; in fact, I knew his was a top of the range Gore-Tex affair. Still, we were making slow progress downwards, with the patient needing frequent support to remain astride the reliable yak, and after what seemed like an eternity, we arrived in Pheriche. This is where the herdsman played a blinder, as he had a chat with a Sherpa mate and managed to get us bunks in a refuge for the night. More money changed hands. Laying the Swede down, he seemed on better fettle already, and more compos mentis. Time for a kip myself.

Next day, with the sun splitting the skies, and knowing that there was a small medical station run by the Himalayan Rescue Association nearby, we plodded along to their hut and discovered a wonderful American respiratory physician on a sabbatical. Together, we checked the Swede over and gave him a good prognosis, with advice to be careful over the next few days, which he of course completely ignored and shot off back up the mountain! The daft prick had disappeared in a millisecond without even a goodbye!

Oh well, but what the hell had I been playing at last night, gloriously riding to the rescue of an ailing soul? Had I actually helped or simply brought someone down the mountain against his will and with his money. The doctor in the refuge thought I had done the right thing, and in fact wrote to my boss commending the action months later. But looking back, I am not sure and yet again should have probably learnt to engage my brain fully and not dance the 'dance wherever I may be.'

Here is another tale, along similar lines . . .

12

WE ALL HANG BY A THREAD

CIRCA 2000

This February night is seared into my memory as the time I encountered the Grim Reaper and looked him in the eye. This tale takes some believing as well as some telling, so please excuse me if it is a little protracted!

It was a grey, damp, icy cold afternoon in February, and Annie, Juliet, Nick and I were going to see my niece, Gracie, perform at a theatre in Cambridge. Little Hannie was too young for the occasion, and so we asked Joan, our doughty babysitter, to come round for the evening. Joan was no ordinary babysitter. Victorian in her bearing, disciplined in her application, she had learnt how to manage a household when in service with Lord and Lady Astor at St James's Square, London. Joan lived in a dear little cottage up the hill from us, and once she got onto our children's wavelength, good times were had by all. Board games, cards, homework, and night time stories were all up for grabs when Joan came around. If Annie and I were really lucky, the ironing would be polished off to boot! Noteworthy was Joan's reception when we returned home from a night out, in that she would always rally on our entry into the sitting room with a crisply delivered,

'Good evening, Doctor, Annie. Have you had a nice evening?'

'Really good thank you, Joan,' Annie and I would reply politely in unison. This night would be no exception, despite the dramatic circumstances of the evening!

Lying on the edge of The Fens, Cambridge was shrouded in a cold mist that night, and after some difficulties, we found a parking space in a side street next to some gated railings leading to a park. We disgorged from our VW Passat Estate and hurried along to the theatre, meeting up with my father, sister and brother-in-law briefly before the performance commenced. Studying the programme, we excitedly awaited the rise of the curtain, when suddenly there was some commotion in the front row.

A member of the audience had collapsed. I got to my feet with that forceful mixture of anxiety, guilt and vocation. More commotion. I hurried down the aisle to find a sturdy-looking gentleman prone on the floor. With the help of another member of the audience, we rolled him over.

Unresponsive. Not breathing. No pulse.

'Christ he's arrested,' I thought.

Another chap joined me, and then another. We called for help and commenced CPR. The three of us rotated cardiac compressions with the rescue breaths. In those days, the ratio of compressions to breaths was 15:2, and you had to get a move on, with nearly two compressions a second. We had regular CPR training in the health centre, where it was suggested that we quietly sing 'Nellie the Elephant' to keep up the required rate;

nowadays, the suggested rate has increased, and we are encouraged to sing 'Staying Alive' by the Bee Gees! With no community defibrillator forthcoming, we kept going, and going . . .

'Nellie the Elephant packed her trunk . . . ,' I sang under my breath.

'Where are those fucking paramedics and ambulance crew?' I thought.

'Nellie the Elephant packed her trunk' . . .

'Where have the paramedics got to?' I enquired.

We kept going, rotating between us, as chest compressions are exhausting. Eventually, I saw in my peripheral vision the green uniforms of the ambulance crew, and carefully we handed the resuscitation over to them. The defibrillation pads were applied and required joules administered. Bam! Activity, real activity on his ECG. Relief and disbelief. We may just have pulled this resus off! He was transported swiftly to Addenbrooke's, where it was rumoured he survived. Remarkable, as survival from cardio-pulmonary resuscitation in the community to successful discharge from hospital varies from a paltry 2% to a more encouraging 12% (*Emerg Med J*, Jan 2012).

Grouped together in front of the stage in a shell-shocked huddle, my two comrades and I deliberated on the next course of action. Two GPs and a pathologist high on adrenaline and feeling like a resuscitation dream team. We quickly asked the gentleman's family before they left for the hospital whether they were happy for the performance to proceed, and upon their assent, we suggested a short break before the audience took to their seats again. The play resumed, but by now Nick and Juliet were wilting, and so at the interval we took our leave of the family and left. Walking back to the car, it dawned on me that my bladder was bursting.

'I am just going through that gate into the park for a tink, Pom. I won't be a minute.'

Through the gate, turning right a few steps, and then . . .

I stepped into a void. I was falling, falling far enough for me to think

'Oh my God, this is going to hurt.'

But no. Woosh!

I was in water, ice cold water and going down, down to the bottom of a murky lagoon. I could feel a sandy floor with my feet and pushed up. Like a bobbing cork, I breached the surface and inhaled. Air.

I was swimming now, and with the cold temperature slamming into my consciousness, I remembered the short survival times of the merchantmen torpedoed in the arctic convoys of WWII.

'Where am I? How do I get out of this cold, nightmarish place? If I hang around in here, this is game over! The merchantmen only had about four minutes!'

Having gathered my thoughts, I swam to the side, where there was a high retaining wall, which looked insurmountable.

I'm trapped in this watery grave. I have only got four minutes.

I had to pull myself up and out but knew my first attempt would be the most likely to succeed before my strength evaporated. I grabbed the wall and to this day do not quite understand how I levered myself out of that place and flopped onto the side. I stood exhausted, staggered to the car and on opening the door heard gasps from my assembled family.

'Andrew, what happened?' enquired Annie.

'Dad,' from the back seat.

I had left my family a slightly dishevelled, clapped-out GP and returned some time later a very wet, dishevelled GP covered in green slime and weed, with a face even more Halloween-like than usual!

We careered out of Cambridge at quite a lick, desperate to get back home and into the warm. Flash! The car was illuminated in a burst of halogen light. Our strange night had just deteriorated further with the visual announcement of a speed camera and the promise of another speed awareness course. This was the final straw, although they do say bad luck comes in threes.

Home at last. Now I just needed to negotiate going upstairs and into the bath without Joan clapping her eyes on the damp ghoulish figure I had mutated into. No such luck, as Joan happened to be in the hall when we turned the key, and on our entry into the house, she enquired without a flicker.

'Good evening, Doctor, Annie. Have you had a good evening?'

Call it training, call it discipline, but it took some doing on Joan's behalf to ignore the bog monster standing in front of her and carry on with her normal enquiry. Carry on she did, however, and all I can say is, good old Joan; Lady Astor would have felt reassured by her sense of decorum that night!

During a hot bath of thermonuclear proportions followed by a hot toddy in bed, I reflected on the tenuous nature of our lives. For much of my existence, I had cruised along with the notion that life was a permanent fixture and I could cheat death. I had intermittent brushes with The Reaper in my job, but on this occasion and on this night, making his acquaintance had become deeply personal, and not to my liking. At what age do we come to realise that life is a gift, to be treasured on a daily basis? In this regard, a cold night in February was part of my coming of age, with two stark reminders that we all hang by a thread.

13

DIAMOND DUST TO STARDUST

CIRCA 2000

A baking hot summer, 1976, in my late teens. I reach for the brown album cover, take out the plain white paper sleeve and put the vinyl on the turntable. *Blow by Blow* by Jeff Beck. I skip the early tracks and drop the stylus bang onto the start of 'Diamond Dust.' Addiction takes many forms, and I was hooked, marvelling at the keyboards and orchestration by one Max Middleton. Six years later, Annie and I are sitting on a £7 plastic sofa, listening to *Grace and Danger* by John Martyn in the lounge of our carrstone cottage in Norfolk. Who is on keyboards on 'Sweet Little Mystery'? Max Middleton. A few years later, I am at the Ipswich Regent watching Chris Rea and looking down from the circle wondering who the keyboard player is. Max Middleton, again augmenting a soundtrack to my youth. *On the Beach*. These were the days before the internet, and so any questions surrounding Mr Middleton the person, the keyboard player, remained just that: questions. An unresolved mystery and my own personal Searching for Sugarman.

It was a hard surgery on a damp Tuesday morning. I had a long list of complicated patients relentlessly requesting definite solutions to difficult problems. Surgeries can vary a lot in their challenge, depending on the age and personality of the patients, and complexity and number of the problems presented. Sometimes, it is possible to fly through the list of patients, and sometimes it is like wading through treacle. I was deep into the sticky stuff this day. Towards the end of the surgery, and in need of oxygen, I saw a new patient on the list with a name I recognised from days gone by, Max Middleton. My memory chimed in. No, it couldn't be, could it? No way! I called through the next patient, and in walked this cheerful chap wearing a white Fedora, looking about the right age. All circumspection and professional communication skills flew out of the window when I blurted out in my excitement,

'Morning, my name is Dr Yager, Andrew. Are you by any chance Max Middleton, the keyboard player?'

'Yep, that's me,' he replied guardedly, probably thinking, 'I came in for medical help, and this buffoon is going to ask for an autograph!'

Wow, thirty years of musical nostalgia sitting right in front of me. My day was suddenly sprinkled with stardust and an enigma resolved.

Now, I had better not go any further with this stream of consciousness without trying to explain what I am rabbiting on about when using the term stardust. Well, it is patient contact that gives a fleeting insight into behaviour or personal history, a slice of information passed on, shared humour, a twinkle in the eye, or a general ambience that enriches the soul of the listener.

Having this contact is a privilege, is uplifting, and enhances the job satisfaction of a GP enormously, but it can only occur when not crippled by time pressure, clinical anxiety and workload. I am also not so naive as to think that all patients fit this mould, as there are a significant number of people who for one reason or another can be very demanding and suck the life blood out of the stoutest GP. For me on this Tuesday morning, however, my life was energised by touching base with the music of my youth, and as I get nearer to retiring, I have learnt to appreciate these nourishing episodes more and more. Such occurrences occur unexpectedly out of the blue from individuals of all shapes, sizes and ages.

In a different week, we had seven-year-old Harry burst through my door, followed hotfoot by his mum declaring in an earnest, deep voice that his ear was sore. In fact, his ear was very, very, very sore and he had come to get it fixed. Part of the delight in seeing Harry was the laughter he engendered in his mother, who obviously rejoiced in his amusing behaviour. In turn, she gave him the confidence, through her loving, protective cloak, to be his own steadfast, comedic self. Then, in came Sally, a police inspector, who during the course of our consultation briefly updated me with a startling intensity and piercing clarity on 'county lines,' exploitation of children and the extent of the drug problem in rural areas. Inspirational Tony, in his 80s with the life force of a man half his age, talked of his desire to get home as soon as possible and bake his annual

35 apple pies for the freezer. Nagin, an IT engineer with the council, quietly entered my consultation room late on the Thursday afternoon, and through his calm, courteous, considered and kindly manner provided an unexpected balm for my frayed nerves. Finally, there was lovely Juliet in her 90s, with a winning smile, soft Scottish lilt and slight memory loss, who charmed me into roaring home from visiting her and announcing to Annie that I had met the most wonderful patient. It was no coincidence that the stardust that touched me that day resulted in our firstborn being called Juliet.

So, surprise, surprise, general practice has interpersonal relationships at its core. Sometimes sweet, sometimes bitter and in turn interesting, challenging, uplifting and enraging, all encountered over the years as doctor and patient slowly age together. I find people interesting and found this aspect of the job rewarding and enriching. I am not alone in this appreciation of these bursts of interpersonal enjoyment, as when on courses and at meetings I have heard numerous health professionals of all persuasions offer up similarly deep, personal and poignant tales. As time marches on, however, I find that the clarity of these ephemeral interpersonal sprinklings of stardust dissipate in the memory. Fortunately, at least where Max Middleton is concerned, I have tucked away in a large wooden box in my attic a vinyl collection where the brown album cover, with the white sleeve, still resides in pride of place. Diamond Dust.

14

SATURDAY

CIRCA 2000

'I told myself that I was going to live the rest of my life as if it were a Saturday.' If this maxim from some know-it-all is true, then I am in for a pretty rough ride. Let me explain.

Shuffling bleary-eyed into the surgery first thing, I was greeted by stalwarts Shirley in reception and dispenser Pauline, ready for action and accustomed to the vagaries of a small team of staff dealing with patient problems varying from the mundane through to the serious. It was not the mundane through to the serious, however, that indelibly burnt this Saturday into our collective memories. It was the chaos, the general level of unbridled relentless calamity that made its mark on this particular Saturday.

Without further ado, we started on the list of patients sitting in the waiting room, including the usual mix of people with urgent problems and needing to see a doctor, people home for the weekend and needing to see a doctor, people unable to attend during the week and needing to see a doctor, and those that had made the common but irritating mistake of running out of medication and needing to see a doctor. A pick-and-mix bag of human concern played out in general practices the length and breadth of the country.

My second patient had a cough and was worried he might be developing a chest infection. We were just getting going when the phone rang.

'Pauline here. I have put Rita in the treatment room, as she has just appeared in the waiting room with heart palpitations, and I think you need to see her now.' Pauline was an experienced straight-talking dispenser of long standing, and when she said 'now,' she meant 'Yesterday.'

Apologising to the coughing patient in front of me, and indicating that I would return soon, I hurried round to Rita lying pale and slightly breathless on the treatment room couch. We talk, and a simple feel of her pulse confirms a rate of 160. Fast for Rita when exercising, and really fast for Rita when lying supine and inert on the treatment room couch. I wheel the ECG over, attach the electrodes and make a recording that indicates Rita's heart has entered into an aberrant rhythm called a supraventricular tachycardia. Not immediately life threatening but in need of urgent treatment. There are certain first aid measures called vagal manoeuvres that stimulate the vagus nerve, causing the heart to slow. The meaning of vagus derives from the Latin for wandering, as this long nerve starts its journey from the medulla of the brain stem, down through the neck, into the thorax and thence into the abdomen, supplying several organs along the way. Stimulate the vagus somewhere along its meandering journey by gagging, coughing, bearing down and pressing on the side of the neck below the jawline and the heart slows. The latter, called carotid sinus massage, was my go-to manoeuvre, and of course on this Saturday of Saturdays it failed miserably. It did not take a rocket scientist to ascertain, on feeling Rita's pulse, that she was still clapping along at 160.

Before Rita and I could discuss the next course of action, Shirley was standing next to me and whispering into my ear, 'I have just taken a garbled call from a panic-stricken mum who says her child has fallen downstairs! I managed to get the name and address before she rang off.'

'OK, I know where that is,' I replied, and on retreating out of the door with Shirley, I muttered, 'Can you get a 999 ambulance for Rita here.'

With the bedside manner of a concrete brick, I shouted over my shoulder, 'Don't worry, Rita, you will be fine; Shirley is getting an ambulance for you. I am afraid I have another emergency.' I was off. I am not sure how fast bats are supposed to leave their eyrie in hell; however, your average bat would have struggled to catch up with me on this day. As to the patient with the cough languishing in my consulting room and consigned to that particular mind-numbing form of waiting room history experienced by us all, he stood no chance in this particular race.

All sorts of medical emergencies played across my mind whilst wheeling my VW Polo around the Monza-like circuit of Suffolk byroads. Severe head injury to neck fracture, via a meagre limb fracture all reared their spectral heads during my short, frenzied journey.

I chose the main door of the cottage, and clunking across the threshold with my bags, I was greeted by the serene scene of a young mum reading to her five-year-old son. 'What happened?' I asked.

'Oh, Simon here fell downstairs from top to bottom and appears fine,' replied the mum as casually as casual can be.

'What, no injuries? We had better check him over even so.'

Amazingly, a check on Simon revealed that mum's assertion was correct. Simon was fine, and just as I was about to clarify any safeguarding issues the phone rang in the kitchen. The mum answered and returning in a jiffy said, 'It's for you doctor!' This was before the days of the ubiquitous mobile.

'Hello, it's me, Shirley, again. You need to get back here as soon as. There has been a crash in the health centre car park,' and with that she hung up. I was stunned but determined to finish one job before moving on. I returned to mum and was quickly satisfied that I had covered all of the possibilities and ramifications of a fall down the stairs. I was off again in my trusty chariot. Monza in reverse, and on two wheels, as the green of the countryside flashed by once again; my grip on the wheel matched only by the pressure on the accelerator and the set of my jaw.

Careering into the car park, I was greeted by a remarkable sight. There in front of me was the standard NHS ambulance I had asked Pauline to request; box-like and reassuring with its logos, blue lights and yellow flashing. Hang on, something is wrong here. Impaled into the flank of the ambulance was a pea green Ford Mondeo, with the ambulance resembling more crushed Coke can than roving apple crate. Near the billowing rear doors of the ambulance was Rita on a gurney, wide-eyed and wan, having been on the trolley in the ambulance when the car struck. The sudden shock of electrical cardioversion can be used to reverse a supraventricular tachycardia; however, in this case study of one, the arrival of a Ford Mondeo into Rita's treatment space did nothing to improve her heart rate. Rita was alive but stirred and shaken to the core, with a heart rate still rumbling on at around 160.

My attention was then drawn away from the ambulance to a man sitting hunched on the low health centre fencing, clutching a nebuliser mask to his face. It was Don, the driver of the pea green Mondeo, with compression for the nebuliser provided by a paramedic operating a foot pump, hands on hips and a remarkably relaxed mien. Rushing to the surgery with an acute exacerbation of chronic obstructive airways disease, Don had completely misjudged his entry into the car park and barrelled into the side of the ambulance, rendering it unroadworthy. Another vehicle or van, as the paramedics like to call them, was on the way. The flotsam and jetsam of medical demand and subsequent carnage was mounting up. Two ambulances, with two patients in the car park, one waiting room full of patients booked in and wanting to be seen on time, a poor chap with a cough still beached in my consulting room, and requests for home visits later on mounting up. I did not know where to start, and 'when do I finish' was banished to my subconscious, as the only way to deal with disorder on this scale was to sequentially and thoroughly sort out each problem in turn. The paramedics would take Rita to hospital in the second van. First, I would sort out Don's chest in the health centre and get him home somehow whilst another paramedic extricated his car from their ambulance. I would then finish seeing the poor chap with the cough in my room and then get started on the queue in the waiting room. The visits could be left to the afternoon, as none of them were urgent.

Unbelievably, this rudimentary plan proceeded smoothly, apart from the small matter of Don's return home. The architect of much of that day's mayhem did not want to play ball, as concerned about leaving his car in the car park, Don insisted on driving his bashed-up Mondeo home.

So, having assessed and treated him in the health centre, I was then leaning through the passenger side window of his crumpled Mondeo, trying to dissuade him from driving. Don gunned the engine, obviously keen to move on. Then, to my horror, I noticed the portable oxygen cylinder on the driver's seat, as he then strapped the attached mask to his face, reminiscent of a certain Spitfire ace. With a nasal cheerio, Don waved me goodbye, hand raised aloft Battle of Britain style: Douglas Bader meets breathless Mondeo man. Oh my God, I thought, this cannot be happening, but happen it did, wild horses and all. I stood stunned as the pea green car chugged out of the car park, down the lane and away over the horizon. My futile attempts to stop him were in vain. All I could do now was hope that he made it home and ring him later to check on his safe return.

Of course, the old maxim 'This day will end' rang true. I eventually returned home in the evening, following some sterling help from Shirley and Pauline, who stayed way beyond their regular hours. I had received a heavy dose of patience from the poor chap with the chest infection holed up in my consulting room for a couple of hours and later, yet again, from wonderful Annie and the children!

Now, normally I love Saturdays, and in this sense Chip Gaines, the progenitor of the quote at the start of this story, has a point. However, I would not want to repeat this particular Saturday any day soon, let alone every day. So, Chip, you are very welcome to visit Botesdale anytime, help with a run of Saturday surgeries, and then decide how you feel about the quote.

15

THE PRICE OF LOVE

2002

Love is priceless, or so the saying goes. Sunday evenings were a struggle when on call over a weekend, and not the ideal time to reflect on the nature of true love. Tiredness was creeping in, with the certain knowledge that a partners' meeting and surgeries awaited next day, before the arrival of Monday evening and a time to relax. Despite these drawbacks, my reverie would be lifted when a house call and a physical manifestation of love was revealed, in all its priceless glory!

Miss Dawson was on the phone, asking me to visit her friend, who was ill in bed with a possible urinary tract infection. The call was not an emergency, but the evening was creeping on and so I went straight away, informing Annie that I would not be long.

Arriving at the house, Miss Dawson, in her mid-70s, greeted me at the door, smartly dressed in a skirt and cardigan, with a searching face and pretty pale blue eyes enhanced by large reading glasses. Without further ado, she efficiently took me upstairs to her friend, who was resting in bed, in the spare room. The friend did indeed have a urinary tract infection, confirmed by a thoughtfully presented specimen. I was able to offer some antibiotics from my bag. Clunking down the stairs with my cases, I noted the wonderful artwork adorning the hall and staircase. Miss Dawson was waiting at the bottom of stairs.

'How is she, Doctor?'

'As you thought, she has a urine infection; she needs to increase her intake of clear fluids and take these antibiotics.'

After further explanation regarding fluids, paracetamol and urine results, I bent down to pick up my bags. Despite the ticking clock, I could not resist returning to the artwork.

'You have some lovely artwork in the house, Miss Dawson,' I declared breezily, juggling my belongings and fishing for an interesting insight.

'Thank you. Do you like art?'

'Yes, I love art, but I don't know much about it.' More fishing!

'Ah, these paintings are all lovely, but my favourite work of art is in my bedroom,' she said firmly, as if a decision had been made, the Rubicon crossed. 'Would you like to see it?'

I had told Annie that I would not be too long, but there was a direction in Miss Dawson's voice that made me dump my bags in the hall and return upstairs, following in her wake. Something special was afoot. Her bedroom was small, and there, above her bed, was an oil painting in a nondescript dilapidated white frame, pitted with woodworm in the bottom right corner. It was an Impressionist scene.

Pointing at the picture, she asked. 'Do you recognise the artist?'

I recognised the Parisian scene, the immediacy of the figures, but not believing what was in front of my eyes, I offered a vague reply.

Miss Dawson came to my rescue, 'It's Renoir, Auguste Renoir.'

Maybe to assuage my shocked state, Miss Dawson then proceeded to let me into her heart and tell me the story of how a genuine Renoir worth millions was hanging in her bedroom, on a Sunday evening on call!

Near the beginning of hostilities in World War II, Miss Dawson signed up and was subsequently stationed in East Anglia. There she met and fell for a young European aristocrat, who had fled the continent in a hurry with two of his family's heirlooms. A Persian rug, sold initially to finance his journey across Europe, and a painting carried in his suitcase, in order to facilitate his relocation on foreign shores. Soon after arriving in England, he signed up with the RAF, subsequently becoming a pilot in bomber command. Chance led him to Miss Dawson, and a wonderful wartime romance blossomed. As their relationship, and the risks associated with his service, intensified, he gave her the picture as a measure of his love.

Tragically, he was killed, leaving Miss Dawson bereft, with the Renoir embodying the life and soul of her one true love. To her, it was not the value of the painting but the memory of the young airman she loved. She could not sell it or change its character in any way, even the bland white frame. Sensibly, she did take it for authentication in Bond Street, London and lifting the picture deftly from the wall, in an action I got the feeling she had done a thousand times before, she showed me the dealer's certificate. I was entranced, excited and felt enormously privileged to be given this heart-rending insight into the measure of her love and attachment to the picture. There was something in her telling of the affair that led me to believe that few people had been given access into this area of her life. Swiftly the painting was returned to its rightful place, and we descended the staircase with little more conversation, except gratitude for the viewing, and further advice for her friend.

Over the years, I began to doubt the veracity of this story, and as the clarity of the event clouded slightly with time, its magnitude intensified in my mind. Was my vivid imagination playing tricks again? Did that really happen? Was I a member of a fortunate few?

I only met Miss Dawson once more, years later, making two meetings in our doctor–patient relationship in total. The second time I was called to her house, she was lying downstairs on a hospital bed, seemingly non-responsive but not in pain. She was terminally ill with hours left to live. I quietly checked she was stable, and as I was about to leave, she opened her eyes, focussed her attention with a weak but charming smile enhanced by the same pale blue eyes and asked quite clearly,

'Do you remember the painting?'

'Of course I remember the picture, Miss Dawson' I stuttered, amazed that she had regained consciousness, knew my voice and was able to speak.

With a weak smile, she shut her eyes again, and that was it. With five words, she had confirmed my memory, affirmed our shared connection, and uttered her final words to me. I left the house with more questions than answers, but the magic of the doctor–patient relationship resounded in my heart with the knowledge that for some fortunate people love is priceless, however short lived.

16

NURSE, THERE'S A GORILLA ON THE WARD!

2002

This is a tale of brushing shoulders with venerated and distinguished medical academics and administrators in Addenbrooke's Hospital one week, to being caught in fancy dress in the same institution the next. Hero to zero within a week!

I was involved with running the postgraduate GP training scheme for West Suffolk. As part of this role, we had to inspect other establishments to ensure that teaching and training standards were being adhered to. On this occasion, the care of the elderly department at Addenbrooke's Hospital, Cambridge was being scrutinised by an inspection team that included yours truly. The NHS thrives on its inspections and meetings, and so on this Wednesday in spring, fifteen clinicians and administrators sat around the large oak table in the Hospital boardroom to discuss teaching standards. Whether this was a good use of time and clinical workforce I am not so sure; however, everyone was very respectful and politely tolerated the scruffy, and slightly thorny, GP who had blown in from the sticks. I enjoyed the attention, the lively debate and the feeling of being close to the corridors of power, in a miasma of vain self-congratulation. At the end of the day, the hospital chief executive bade me farewell with a beaming smile, in an apparently sincere and cheerful expression of thanks for my invaluable contribution to the day and with the hope that we would meet again soon. An enduring friendship? Little did he know!

During the course of this week, a great fishing friend of mine had been admitted to Addenbrooke's Hospital for a liver transplant. Being a haemophiliac, Jonathan had received Factor 8 contaminated with Hepatitis C years ago and following end-stage liver failure was listed for a transplant. Believe it or not, Jonathan was the lucky one, as his brother had contracted HIV through the same process, and died. One of the biggest blunders ever served up by the NHS rumbles on to this day, leaving a dwindling number of surviving haemophiliacs and an increasing number of bereft families in its wake.

Any hospital stay was due to be interminable, and so I resolved, with another friend, Greg, to visit Addenbrooke's and cheer up Jonathan, who was languishing on the ward and awaiting life-saving surgery.

As a junior doctor, I had looked after a lovely lady, Kathy, terminally ill with cancer on the ward. Intermittently, husband Martin would arrive on the ward in fancy dress, and the transformation in the mood on the ward, as well as the smile on Kathy's face, struck a chord with me, which I had not forgotten.

So, Greg and I found ourselves on our way to Addenbrooke's, via a fancy-dress outfitter in Newmarket, dressed as a gorilla and dog. Plastic face and shaggy outfit for Greg, and a tail and a large head with floppy ears for yours truly. Time was short, which is why we had donned our outfits in the shop, making haste to the hospital via the motorway in full attire, without incident.

Now, the visibility in these costumes is not great, and so finding the correct ward, which is challenging at the best of times, was nigh on impossible. The dog and the gorilla ended up blundering around the hospital corridors, amusing some people and terrifying others, in a welter of confusion. Eventually, we careered on to the liver unit, with Greg mistakenly leading the charge on to the female side of the ward as I was slowed to a shuffle by my tail, concertinaed legs and large paws! Just as we realised that we were in the wrong section of the ward, a confused, jaundiced lady with probable hepatic encephalopathy looked up and cried out at the top of her voice,

'Nurse, there's a gorilla on the ward, and it is coming over to me. It's coming to get me!'

Seeing that this scenario could get out of hand, I got Greg to reverse and flee from the ward as fast as our outfits could carry us. Shuffle, shuffle. Slip, slide. Hasta la vista baby!

'Nurse, it's running away. It's escaping. Get after it!'

Concerned that hospital security would be after us, we managed as quickly as possible to find Jonathan, who was sitting on his bed. His hearty laughter on seeing us made our brush with capture worth it. He was keen to get off the ward and venture down to the canteen in the main concourse, meaning we had to retrace our steps gingerly whilst trying vainly to remain as incognito as possible. By now I had the padded dog's head in one hand, in an effort to cool down, and the tail in my other. Oh no! Padded, pawed and shuffling downstairs, I then ran smack bang into the hospital chief executive, who had waved me off the previous week with a show of enduring friendship. Forgetting what a ridiculous sight I looked, and that he would not recognise me let alone remember me, I enquired of the chief executive,

'Hello, how are you?'

'Fine, thank you,' he replied slightly defensively, with a perplexed look on his face.

'Good inspection last week,' I blurted out in an utterly misguided attempt to achieve common ground and strike up a dialogue.

'Er, yes, good thank you,' he said, looking into my beet red beaming face with a dismissive gaze before subsequently shimmying away, no doubt with hospital security now top of his agenda!

I told you it was hero to zero.

We had had to follow the chief executive down the stairs before we could shuffle off into a rambling corridor, where we burst into the hospital canteen in a tide of good humour and laughter. With Jonathan eventually returned to the ward looking a lot more chipper, we departed the hospital with no further hiccups. With us safely back in the black VW Golf on the motorway, I was left to reflect on the day's events in comparison to my previous trip to the teaching wing of Addenbrooke's. My conclusion: there was no comparison. Career progression and moving in academic circles are all very well, but what really makes the world go round and warms the heart is comradeship and the laughter of friends!

Fortunately, Jonathan's liver transplant was a rip-roaring success, and through a vital mix of optimism, steely determination, family support and courage, twenty years later he is still here to share this story; a living, breathing embodiment of the remarkable but error-strewn advancement of medical science. Sadly, the dog and the gorilla have no more ventures in the pipeline. Not too long after this escapade, Greg the gorilla started to struggle with his memory; in his early sixties, he was diagnosed with Primary Progressive Aphasia and lost the ability to speak. For a jovial, kind and witty man of medicine, this was the cruellest of fates. The memories of his laughter and thoughtful disposition, however, live on.

17

CHRISTOPHER COLUMBUS'S
FINAL VOYAGE

2003

'Andrew! Jay and I have been talking, and we have come up with a plan,' suggested Jim, Annie's father, as he came through the door into the kitchen, orthopaedic textbook in hand. It was Christmas Eve in Adelaide Park, Belfast, and I was slightly taken aback, firstly by the urgency in Jim's voice, and secondly by the fact that he was standing in the kitchen for the first time in my experience. We sat down at the table and started to peruse the textbook of orthopaedic operative surgery in detail. This had got to be some plan!

Annie and her mum Joy were enjoying the craic, hovering around the Aga excitedly chatting with our three children, Juliet, Nick and Hannie. We all loved going over to Belfast at Christmas, with the coal fires, endless food and warm cheer. Through force of personality, cheerfulness and common sense, Jim and Joy had managed to raise a family, with five well-adjusted children, during The Troubles in Belfast, which were now entering their final stages. It was definitely a time to make the most of Christmas.

Annie's brother Jay had mentioned that he was struggling with clawing of a couple of his toes, losing his toenails on a regular basis. Jim was an orthopaedic surgeon of international repute, and nearing the end of his clinical work, this was enough for him to jump at the chance to work up a scheme to help Jay.

'Joy and I will come over and stay with you and Pom in Rickinghall this Easter. Jay and Poppy can then come up from London for the operation at the start of the holidays. We'll provide the theatre equipment and then undertake the surgery in your minor operations room in the health centre, Andrew.'

At this, Joy chipped in, with a twinkle in her eye, 'Are you enrolling me as a theatre sister again Jim?'

'Och, you know you are the one and only theatre sister for me, Joy,' Jim said with a wry grin and a chuckle. Carrying on, he ventured, 'How does that sound, Andrew?'

'That sounds great, Jim, just great,' I replied meekly, realising by now that with both my in-laws keen to embark on this madcap venture resistance was futile. On the one hand, I was excited at the thought of seeing everyone over Easter; however, I was not fully convinced that our health centre was the best place to undertake significant orthopaedic foot surgery. Ah well, in for a penny, in for a pound, and at that time on a raucous Christmas Eve, Easter and a surgical risk assessment seemed a long way away! That was it, the die was cast. Easter it was, with Jim and Joy intending to cross the Irish Sea with one major goal in mind. Serious surgery, and in my health centre!

Before I knew it, we were driving through the village to the health centre one evening over the Easter holidays after the normal day's work had finished. Fully gowned, and with Jay on the operating couch, we commenced the surgery with Jim in charge and Joy on sparkling form as the archetypal theatre sister. We made a start using the particular incision discussed at Christmas, and once I heard Jim whistling through his teeth into his mask, I knew all was proceeding smoothly, and he was in the zone. I felt a wave of nostalgia on realising that this would probably be the final time Jim and Joy would work together undertaking the roles they were both trained for. It was a privilege to be present at their last hurrah.

Then, we hit a problem. Scar tissue rendered any attempt to undertake the textbook operation impossible, and from then on, we were in unchartered territory. Jim decided to change tack, clip away some bone and fuse the final joints in the two toes. Things for a while got more difficult, and my wave of nostalgia was replaced with anxiety.

Guardedly, I looked up and saw Jay's jaw clenched tight; the look of horror evident in his eyes as bone fragments spiralled onto the floor. Unbeknown to me, as a child he had been introduced to the notion of a Christopher Columbus operation by his surgeon father. This was an operation where the surgeon sets off into unchartered waters not knowing where they are going or how to get there, if at all! Jay explained afterwards that all he could think of when watching the bone fragments was, 'This is a Christopher Columbus. I'm having a Columbus. This wasn't what we talked about at all!'

So where did this familial voyage of exploration land? I am glad to report that despite one or two changes in tack and a painful initial recovery, the operation was a rip-roaring success, with Jay's toes pain free to this day.

Over the years, I have undertaken quite a lot of minor surgery in our health centre, and as a service for patients it is invaluable. I am more Arthur Ransome than Christopher Columbus, undertaking simple procedures, from removal of sebaceous cysts through to ingrowing toenails, cryotherapy and joint injections. Significant orthopaedic operations, however, on family members, without a known direction of travel, remain firmly off the menu of surgical options, now and for evermore! As for Jim and Joy, this procedure did turn out be their final surgical voyage together, albeit joined in their ventures by family and the ghost of Christopher Columbus himself!

18

COLLEEN

CIRCA 2005

Despite being part of the NHS, general practices are run as self-employed businesses and as such are responsible for the finances, staffing and a multitude of other areas within the practice structure. This gives a degree of autonomy and requires the partners to engage their business brains as well as attend to the medical side of things. Nowadays, the NHS has really improved its training in these matters, with a plethora of leadership courses, financial updates and business training. When I started, we just got on with it, relying on the older, more seasoned partners to steer the ship with the help of a practice manager, and often learning through the bitter pill of experience.

Managing staff relations and human resources was frequently undertaken on a day-to-day basis by the practice manager; however, knotty problems would be brought to a partner's door. When undertaking clinical medicine, one's focus is solely on trying to do the best for the patient, which I was comfortable with. When dealing with colleagues, tensions can arise, which I found more difficult and unsettling. Factor in that most of our staff were also our patients, leading to a doctor–patient, employee–employer melee, it was a human resources perfect storm. A few years ago, I sailed unwittingly into such a situation where the boundaries blurred between patient and colleague, and fortunately by hook and by crook both of us came through the other side to tell the tale. Let me explain . . .

Jill, our previous practice nurse, was retiring to Spain, and having advertised and interviewed for a replacement, we finally settled on Colleen, who joined us from the West Suffolk Hospital. Approachable, excellent with patients and with plenty of clinical nous, Colleen and I settled into a comfortable working relationship, after a slightly shaky start born of the fact that I had probably expected too much too soon from her. Practice nursing is vastly different to hospital nursing and requires a completely different skill set, consequently taking years rather than months to master, with Colleen no exception. As time passed, I increasingly valued Colleen's clinical judgement, her knowledge of our patients on a personal level, and also her kindness and enthusiasm. We became good buddies with a shared ethos of patient care.

One day Colleen popped her head round the door of my consultation room to update me on her own recent admission to hospital with abdominal pain, the cause of which had baffled the admitting surgeons. The only thing amiss was her liver function tests, and after hearing her story on a background of gall bladder surgery, I suggested an ultrasound scan of her abdomen. Quickly completing the form before the next patient, we resolved in our haste to talk again when the scan result returned. A hurried chat, a decision and a scribbled ultrasound referral completed in a flash, with the throng of patients in the morning waiting room never far from the back of our minds.

A relatively short period of time later, a yellow radiology result form landed on my desk with Colleen's name on it and to my horror a result indicating that she had renal cell cancer in one kidney. I broke the news to her and then resolved to get her along the cancer pathway as quickly as possible, with the kidney eventually being successfully removed in Norwich. During our conversations, she was always calm and very courageous, balancing the need for time off with her desire to keep working and undertake the job she was so good at. Somehow, she managed to deal with her fears around her own mortality, her family, friends and future whilst staying at work, where she found solace and support from being around us, her colleagues. Those days are now firmly behind her, I am glad to say; however, when reflecting on those initial conversations, I break out in a cold sweat. At no time did we formerly sit down and undertake a formal medical conversation, examination or treatment plan, with everything done on the hoof in between the next patient. With hindsight, I would have maybe organised things differently in terms of patient–staff–doctor boundaries; however, on this occasion, all's well that ends well, with the storm well and truly behind us! Colleen is a cancer survivor and a brave one at that, and in terms of our employer–employee relationship, she repaid our decision to recruit her, a nurse from the West Suffolk Hospital, a thousand times.

As well as dealing with day-to-day employment issues, it is also really important that the partners set the tone of the practice within the workforce and articulate verbally and in their behaviour the underlying ethos, values and ideals of the organisation. I was very fortunate when joining Botesdale, in that the practice had a proud history of patient-centred care that was second to none, with partners Bill and Rob more than embodying this trait. I was privileged in the fact that I simply had to put my shoulder to the wheel and continue along in the same vein. I did not have to effect positive change or alter practice direction, as the organisation I was joining was supremely functional. Despite the fantastic hand I was dealt, I realised soon enough that keeping the practice patient-focussed, up to date and a source of local pride year in year out takes energy, commitment and the ability to carry the workforce along on the journey. This is a difficult task that must be embraced, as stories abound of GP practices that have slowly gone down the tubes through lack of leadership and clarity of purpose. The expression 'lack of leadership' encompasses a multitude of things; however, employing and sustaining the most suitable and able people can more than make up for other leadership qualities that may be lacking. I look back and think we made some really excellent staff recruitment decisions over the years, with many staying with us for decades. It wasn't always easy;

however, hopefully this process translated into a patient-centred vision of general practice carried forward by the practice workforce, with dear Colleen firmly at the vanguard of a long and proud roll call of individuals.

19

PEARLS OF WISDOM

CIRCA 2005

General practice has a proud tradition of training its new recruits via a one-year placement in a teaching practice. Support, mentorship and education are provided by a trainer, who themselves undergo assessment, education and trainers' group meetings. Botesdale Health Centre was one such practice, with Rob and I the trainers.

Embarking on a future career in general practice, a GP registrar will leave their training practice with a wealth of ideas, experience and knowledge. Some of the most poignant memories of a trainee's time in practice will be the aphorisms and maxims passed on to them by the doctors working in the practice, who will have accumulated a store of knowledge, much of it gleaned from the bitter pill of experience. It is these 'pearls of wisdom' and tricks of the trade that interested me.

In an attempt to allow these aphorisms to see the light of day, I wrote to all the trainers in our training group in 2005, asking them to consider their own 'pearls of wisdom.' After a considerable gestational period, we were delighted when the twelve training practices in our group generated over 200 responses from over

113

thirty trainers. Further discussion ensued, enabling us to categorise and analyse the responses, leading to a small printed booklet intended to be educational as well as thought-provoking. I have lifted many but by no means all of the aphorisms from this booklet and listed them in the original categories used: communication, attitude, time management, clinical banana skins, caring for oneself. I have left the pearls in their unabridged form, without further comment, as I want the reader to make what they will of them. Not set in tablets of stone and open to dispute, I hope they are an interesting insight into the inner sanctum of the GP consulting room, around the time of the millennium.

Communication

- During the consultation – listen, listen and listen again; the patient will generally spill the beans in the first few lines – so shut it! After you have said the introductions and formalities, stay quiet for the first two minutes.
- Make sure you know why the patient is seeing you.
- The unasked question is like a broken pencil – pointless.
- Patients usually consult with concerns not symptoms.
- Good telephone advice can take just as long as a face-to-face consultation. Follow the same consultation guidelines.
- When you haven't a clue what is going on, ask the patient – but learn to phrase it properly.

114

- Not all problems need to be resolved in one consultation but ideally should be acknowledged.
- Be clear on what information the patient wants before giving any out.
- Keep it simple – too many words from the GP can add up to a load of nonsense.
- When managing elderly, frail, confused patients, maintain good communication with the relatives. Phone them if in doubt.
- If you are offering reassurance, you must know exactly what the patient is concerned about.
- Be clear about follow up. Never say 'see how you go.'

Attitude

- The patient is usually right.
- Most people are reasonable and understanding.
- Patients respond more positively and use services more reasonably if treated with kindness and dignity.
- Patients rarely sue doctors they like.
- Be nice to people – especially pathologists!
- A kindness is always repaid. Unpleasantness is always repaid tenfold.
- Always treat a patient as you and your family would like to be treated.
- Do not make jokes at the patient's expense.
- Do not get angry with patients. If you do, you make presumptions and lose your clinical edge.

- Honesty is a virtue. Confess lack of knowledge or mistakes. Patients appreciate it.
- If you don't know the answer, inform the patient; don't be embarrassed to admit that you don't know; to look things up during a consultation; to change your mind about a management decision.
- Medical paternalism and arrogance are dead in today's society. Today's doctor needs humility, a sense of humanity and, where possible, a sense of humour.
- When a consultation is going badly, acknowledge it and enlist the patient's help in working out why.
- Agree first, negotiate later. If the patient is demanding a treatment or visit, it often helps to agree to their request first and then negotiate later. If you say no before they have got their demands off their chest, it can get their back up.
- Demands have more than one reason. For instance, the patient may be very stressed and worried; under pressure from family and friends; habitually demanding.
- Run towards your troubles, rather than away from them.
- Never give up on the patient.
- Confront your mistakes.

Time management
- If you are running late, don't panic. Give every patient the time they deserve, and on the whole other patients won't mind.

- Never put off what you know has to be done in a consultation; do it now, as you will be just as busy, if not busier, next time, and you will wish you had done it the first time.

- The difference between doing a good job and a bad job is usually only a short amount of time.

- Men in particularly don't dress quickly when you are talking to them. After examining them, say 'We'll chat when you are dressed,' and they then dress like grease lightning. Saves time.

- If you have to do a cremation form at the undertakers, park where the hearse normally parks. You then get prompt attention and save time.

- Never touch a piece of paper or computer file more than once. Don't put things away that you think you might need to look at another time, as they will certainly end up being thrown away in six months, without being looked at again.

- Do one thing at a time.

- If you are always running late, you need shorter surgeries, or longer appointments, or both.

- Don't let junior colleagues or staff delegate upwards. Help them to solve their problems themselves.

- Make sure you see the bottom of your in tray at least once a week.

- Make the telephone work for you. Work out a policy for telephone contacts.

Avoiding clinical banana skins

- The physician entertains the patient whilst nature affects the cure. *This is a rework of a quote by Voltaire.*

- When you look out of the window in the morning and see a big bird, it may be a golden eagle but is more likely to be a pigeon: common things occur commonly.

- Beware of odd symptoms and signs. Keep scratching around until you get the answer, or the patient gets better. Remember that rare conditions occur more regularly than you think because there are a lot of different rare conditions.

- Follow your intuition and listen to your waters. If your intuition tells you that something is wrong, you ignore this feeling at the patient's peril.

- Situations evolve, and time is usually on your side, but be careful.

- The history is very important in general practice ophthalmology. Do not rush to pick up the ophthalmoscope, but always check the visual acuity.

- If you do not know what is wrong with a patient, a good place to start is to dip their urine and check their temperature and pulse.

- If an elderly man complains of urinary symptoms, remember to feel the abdomen for an enlarged bladder, as it is easy to miss chronic urinary retention.

- Remember that recurrent urinary infections in the elderly can herald serious underlying disease and may require further investigation.
- When dealing with small children, always believe the mother's intuition.
- When treating sick children, remember that children can deteriorate very rapidly and therefore have a low threshold for reviewing, revisiting, or admitting to hospital.
- Ask a young child with a sore ear which ear he or she would like the doctor to look at first. Then when they indicate a particular ear, consent is given, and the examination will proceed more smoothly.
- If a patient depresses you, it may be because the patient is depressed.
- When listening to a chest, always remember the 'silent conditions' such as a collapsed lung or fluid on the lung.
- When a woman of childbearing age presents with abdominal pain and/or vaginal bleeding, always think ectopic pregnancy.
- If you are asked to prescribe a new drug you do not know much about, always look it up first in the British National Formulary.
- Always observe the 'three strikes rule.' If the patient keeps calling you out, you may be missing something and so be prepared to admit them to hospital on the third call and have a good reason for not doing so on the second.
- Check your bag before going out on visits.

Caring for self

- Don't worry about things that haven't happened.
- You are no good to anybody unless you look after yourself.
- Be grateful for what you have got, and enjoy the simple things in life.
- Every single moment in life is of importance.
- Learn to tolerate your uncertainty.
- The art of surviving in general practice is to learn how to take the short cuts safely.
- When things get tough, take a deep breath and keep going. Your surgery will finish.
- Be flexible, embrace change and keep learning.
- Can you think of a job you would rather do? If not, stop grumbling.
- There is no point in worrying all night or weekend about having not acted. It is better to get home half an hour late and then forget about things, rather than get home half an hour early and worry.
- Keep a file of all the nice cards and letters that patients send you. When you are having a tough day or a patient complains, it helps a great deal to refer to the 'good feeling file,' in order to maintain a proper sense of balance.
- When you return from holiday, always know when your next holiday is going to be.

And finally . . .

- Because of the breadth of general practice, it is far more difficult being a good general practitioner than a hospital specialist. The specialist can close his or her mind to large areas of medicine and say 'that is not my field.' The general practitioner, however, has to know something, and often quite a lot, about most areas of medicine.

- Being a good GP is difficult (and virtually impossible in today's NHS).

- Beware of aphorisms – including this one, naturally! The diversification of general practice will always provide an example to disprove any generalisation you care to make, usually at an inconvenient or crucial moment.

- A doctor who offers up a lot of aphorisms is probably becoming a middle-aged bore!

20

A SELFLESS SOUL

CIRCA 2008

There are some people who are intrinsically and intuitively adept at caring for others: life's natural-born carers. It requires a skill set which includes an ability to work hard, intelligence, diligence, selflessness, and an attention to detail, especially if things go awry. Harry was such a person, lovingly looking after wife Gertrude during her latter years of infirmity. He was a quiet, wiry man of the soil, with a shock of white hair, engaging eyes and a kind, generous smile. Gertrude was a chatty, charming woman, with a ready laugh and a twinkle in the eye. Together as octogenarians they led a quiet life, diminished somewhat by Gertrude's restricted mobility.

One day in early summer, I was called to their house, as Gertie was struggling to stand, having migrated slowly from walking stick, to frame and now reluctantly to wheelchair. This is a journey many of us make, and despite improved strategies to keep us mobile, including physiotherapy and occupational therapy, arresting and dealing with this decline can be problematic. All of the household chores, and much of the lifting and mobilisation of Gertrude, were undertaken by Harry in his usual steadfast way. During the visit, it was evident that the situation was not ideal, leaving me feeling slightly overwhelmed by Gertrude's infirmity and the realisation that there was no quick and easy fix. Determined to be positive, I went through a plan and hopefully provided some encouragement to Gertrude. There was no doubt, though, that my solutions felt like papering over the cracks, with a situation that could unravel at a moment's notice. Both Gertrude and Harry were not in their first flush, living in circumstances that would test people half their age. The physical and mental stresses and strains of infirmity can be enormous. How would this charming elderly couple cope? On bidding my goodbyes, Harry was showing me out of the door when I glimpsed the back garden entirely devoted to fruit and vegetables. Out of the corner of my eye, I saw carefully managed fruit trees and fruit cages, encircled by a profusion of vegetables in neatly tended rows.

'Your garden is impressive, Harry.' I needed to communicate with Harry, the person and the carer, gauge his take on the situation, with his garden being as good a place to start as any.

'Thank you. Are you interested in gardening, Doctor? I can let you have a look if you like?'

No, not really, I thought. I am rushed off my feet! My rational brain was telling me to press on; but my heart was telling me that I wasn't finished here and to stay awhile.

'OK, Harry,' I muttered, clutching my silver examination bag in an effort to remain workmanlike and pushed for time.

As well as being impressed by Harry's horticultural knowledge and skills, I was mindful of the time and energy needed to cultivate such a garden. If I had been in Harry's position, I would have been struggling, physically and psychologically, to cope with Gertrude. I would be anxious, deflated and diminished. Just how did he do all of this? How did he manage to keep smiling and remain so calm?

Slowly we strolled along the rows and around the perimeter of the large garden, discussing the whys and wherefores of, and plans for, his garden. I was mesmerised by Harry's diligence and tranquillity. I was even considering discarding my examination bag for a while!

Eventually, we arrived at some greenhouses. Harry stopped and enquired with a smile,

'Would you like to see a couple of my friends?'

Not really knowing what was on offer, I was intrigued, and on crossing the threshold into the greenhouse, there before me in a large wooden pen were two small tortoises.

Harry bent over to pick one of them up. 'This one is the oldest, and I have had her from the age of eight! My mum got her from the pet shop when I was a small boy.' I couldn't contain the surprise in my voice. 'Harry, you mean to say you have looked after this tortoise for 78 years?' I exclaimed, struck by the thought of this man lovingly looking after this small creature for so long. Food, water, cleaning and preparing for hibernation, week in week out, for the guts of a century!

'More or less, yes,' he replied with typical modesty.

'What is her name?'

'Sorry, I never got round to giving her a name.' Again, I was shocked; however, it subsequently occurred to me that in caring for these creatures Harry did not need to humanise them. Quietly looking after them to keep them healthy and safe was enough.

After a while, I took my leave and while driving home reflected on Harry; he was a born carer and had nurtured his nameless tortoises though love, diligence and an attention to detail. Likewise, his fruit and vegetable garden was the stuff of dreams. My concerns about how he would manage Gertrude's infirmity were misplaced. At this point in time, Harry had ample gas in the tank to cope, and as long as he was physically able he would tenderly look after his wife to the best of his ability, with a ready smile and a quiet determination. Selfless hard work, tenderness and sacrifice were part and parcel of this man's soul, and as it turned out this couple coped well together for many months, without a hitch. Once a carer, always a carer!

Interestingly enough, I wonder if I would have arrived at the same firm conclusion of a stable, rock-solid home situation without the insights into the garden and tortoises. Who knows; however, what I would say is that I was surer footed in my decision-making with this information to hand. Recently in primary care, via a combination of a wider workforce and remote working, GP home visiting is on the decline. Under the guise of workforce efficiency, this decline is sure to gather steam, and I cannot help but wonder if the absence of rich personal insights provided by GP home visiting will be to the ultimate detriment of primary care.

Finally, whilst gaining consent for this story, I made contact with the household, discovering that, sadly, Gertrude is no longer with us. Harry, however, is now a nonagenarian, still going strong and attending to his strawberries, with both tortoises hot on his heels.

21

BURNOUT AND BUOYANCY AIDES

2008

One of my medical heroes is Dr Clare Gerada, ex-Chair of The Royal College of GPs and long-term campaigner in striving for mental health help for GPs. In a refrain that I will return to again in these essays, Clare states that general practice has become an impossible job with the time limited to 10-minutes for a consultation. Expectation is rocketing, medical complexity is increasing and yet consultation times remain woeful, with GPs living with safety fears, inadequacy and patient disappointment. The result: anxiety and depression in all GP age groups from 27 to 70. Clare, in her inimitable way, has, over the last couple of years, set up a mental health and wellbeing self-referral service dedicated to supporting GPs with their mental health. For years I have envied private counsellors and psychotherapists with their long consultation times, strict client numbers and mandated counselling for themselves, whilst the clapped-out old GP bashes on regardless. Clare is now trying to address this shortfall in professional self-help. I await with interest to see whether she can also do anything about consultation times and patient numbers per day.

As my own general practice career has progressed, I have become more aware of, and interested in, my own mental health. As a newly qualified GP, I felt I was immune to stress, paying very little heed to my own wellbeing; however, as my life got busier and busier, the cracks began to show. New job, growing family, new house requiring renovation, I misguidedly decided to undertake a master's degree. A bridge too far, and a brush with burnout, which I was able to deal with by a slight reduction in clinical commitment and a change in role for a time. It was a close shave which made me realise how GPs need to be very much aware of their own mental state. All GPs are stressed; however, when that stress becomes chronic, with loss of function, burnout is on the horizon. I conceived an analogy where we are on the shores of a lake with the water as a source of comfort as well as danger. All GPs are paddling on the water's edge, splashing, kicking and enjoying the experience of heightened awareness and spirit that a certain degree of stress and sense of vocation can bring. No GP is on the beach sunning themselves! Venture in up to your calves, and wading becomes more sluggish and testing. Up to your hips is harder still, and then up to your chest you are in danger of bobbing under and drowning at a moment's notice. This is the GP who comes into work, experiences the final straw, hits the wall and is off work for months. Factor in the googly ball of the medical complaint or medical litigation and even the sternest individual can be removed at the stumps for a duck.

This problem is not confined to primary care. Recently, I was talking to a normally jovial consultant at our local hospital, who informed me that he and many of his fellow colleagues had at some time in their recent careers considered throwing themselves off the Orwell Bridge near Ipswich, which obviously at the height of 43 metres is a one-way ticket. I am not sure what I found more disconcerting: the fact that many consultants consider suicide or the fact they have discussed a preferred route, the Orwell Bridge. As a junior doctor during training and four weeks into a new hospital job, I walked into ITU and came across a fellow house officer hooked up to a ventilator having taken a near lethal overdose. No one is immune to the effects of stress in the NHS; it can be brutal. The secret is understanding where you are in this watery continuum at all times and taking steps to move into shallower waters or seek a buoyancy aide when in too deep. Learning from these analogies and mixed metaphors was very instrumental in helping me in my career, with Clare's recent GP mental health service a long overdue life raft.

Buoyancy aides can come in all shapes and sizes and are a necessary accessory in all walks of life. On a dog walk one weekend, Bill, my ex-senior partner, pulled up in his Honda, winded the window down and asked if I was going for a walk in the near future. 'It's just that if you are, you may want to consider asking Chris to come along with you.'

As it happens, I was planning to walk along the North Norfolk Coast and so in due course phoned Chris, our local village rector, with an invitation to join me on the trek. The role of a parish priest is not an easy job, with similar stresses and strains to being a village GP:

accountability, perceived moral status, decreasing revenues forcing closures, increasing workload. Seven years is around the time that these factors can start to erode the wellbeing of the average rector, and exacerbated by an infection, Chris was no exception to this rule, resulting in a spell of time off. Hesitantly, Chris agreed to join me on some of my journey, with Barbara, his wife, agreeing to pick him up at the Victoria Pub, Holkham, after a day's walking.

Starting off on our walk, I realised that Chris was quite a chatterbox, and so conversation flowed at a rate of knots, about all sorts. Quickly we arrived at our first pub, The Thornham Lifeboat. I was not sure that beer was the ideal remedy for Chris at this stage; however, I have always loved this pub and as such it was too good an opportunity to miss.

'Fancy a pint, Chris?'

'Why not? It looks to be a Woodforde's pub, so with luck there will be Wherry on tap.'

And sure enough, Wherry was on tap, and in the next pub, the next and the next. By the end of the day, we had walked quite a distance and shared a lot of laughter, fuelled by more than the odd pint. We both enjoyed the experience, and Chris returned home in a slightly better, albeit inebriated, state than when he set off. So, what made this short walk such a positive experience? Well, the ability to share the trials and tribulations of village life and work within a confidential setting, not to mention laughter and a large dose of Woodforde's Wherry! Now, I am not a particularly spiritual person, attending church for weddings, funerals and Christmases only. I do not spend much time thinking about the spiritual world and found Chris's conversation on this realm interesting. I did not necessarily agree with all of his spiritual beliefs; however, I admire anybody who explores their spirituality in its broadest and most benign sense. So what started off as a kindly act ended up being a two-way street, with my wellbeing also enhanced.

So, on returning home, we resolved to undertake a similar venture the following year, with the result that over the last decade we have slowly worked our way along the East Anglian coastline. Norfolk and Suffolk have been completed, with the long, meandering and estuary-filled Essex coastline underway. For Chris, these walks have become an aforementioned buoyancy aide during the last few years of his pastoral life, whereas for me, in the throes of retirement, the goal now is getting around the coastline before decrepitude bites!

So what have I learnt about burnout during my career? Firstly, to acknowledge that no one is immune; to understand where you are in the continuum between stress and burnout; and secondly, to incorporate as many buoyancy aides into day-to-day life as possible. If these fail, then self-refer to the GP mental health service sooner rather than later. Thank you, Clare, for setting this service up. Thank you, Chris, for walking the long walk . . .

22

COMMUNICATION: THE GOOD, THE BAD AND THE UGLY!

VARIOUS DATES

Decision-making comes thick and fast in general practice. It is not rocket science but more about quick-fired intuitive pragmatism, on the back of solid communication. What happens, though, when for one reason or another this communication misfires? Well, here are three such examples, with wildly differing outcomes . . . the good, the bad and the ugly!

The Good

Partner Rob had just started a busy evening surgery when he called Mrs Shaw in from the waiting room. No Mrs Shaw. Unusual.

Mrs Shaw was a very punctual and considerate person who by nature would telephone and cancel any appointment she could not attend. A seed of doubt in Rob's gut forced him to ring Mrs Shaw's home telephone a couple of times. No reply.

As the evening wore on, the kernel of anxiety grew, and with his intuition screaming at him that something was amiss, Rob felt he should drop around to check on her. This was no mean undertaking, as she lived out in the sticks, and he really wanted to return home, see his wife Sue and the children before bedtime, and grab a bite to eat. After a brief pause wrestling with this dilemma, anxiety and intuition won the day over personal comfort and family affairs, and before he knew it, he was on his way to her bungalow.

On arrival, Rob rang the bell several times. No answer. He then heard a plaintiff cry, however, from a bathroom window around the side of the house. To him, it sounded like a cry for help. Having gained access via another utility room window, he found Mrs Shaw trapped in the bath, with the water drained. The bath had been her tomb for two days, and potentially her final resting place. Despite being hypothermic, with a temperature below 35 degrees centigrade, and very stiff, he managed to lift Mrs Shaw from the bath, wrap her in blankets, and arrange for admission to hospital via an ambulance. He stayed with her until the ambulance arrived, during which time she feebly made him promise to feed her cats during her admission!

The following, day Rob scooted into work as usual, sat at his desk and modestly regaled this remarkable story of decision-making and action informed by intuition and tacit knowledge. Not high tech or high profile, and some would say more of a social than a medical problem, but a life saved by a GP thinking holistically and doing his job to the best of his ability, including the feeding of the cats twice daily!

The Bad

It was late on a Bank Holiday Monday afternoon, and an elderly, anxious gentleman with acute abdominal pain was on the phone requesting a visit, sooner rather than later. Dr Tim was busy doing a shift for the GP Out-of-Hours Co-operative, and with calls stacking up, he resolved to visit as soon as he could. A couple of hours later, Tim knocked on the door of the patient's flat, with no answer, no noise from inside, and no response from repeated calls on the landline call-back number. In a repeat of the previous scenario, nothing!

Tim said he had considered the possible causes of this silence, including cardiac arrest, ruptured aortic aneurysm and other life-threatening conditions. Still no answer, and thinking the worst, with no time to lose, the police were summoned, and with a door battering ram in hand, informally known as 'The Big Red Key,' Tim and the police were through the shattered front door in seconds searching the flat for signs of life, or death. Not a soul was in sight!

Feeling flummoxed and tense, and wondering what to do next, they returned outside only for the patient to come sauntering round the corner on his way home from shopping. Eventually, the gentleman was sort of pacified and attended to and a carpenter was called. It seems that he believed Tim wouldn't be visiting for some time and on account of feeling better had gone out to buy some food for tea.

Tim, desperate to get off to the other urgent calls waiting on his list, managed to extricate himself with a cheerful wave, whilst the police shuffled off as well.

Now, I will let the reader decide on the rights or wrongs of this scenario, but suffice it to say that I suspect the next time the gentleman makes a visit request he will not leave his premises without cancelling the visit! Tim acted on the available information, made a decision and acted quickly, maybe too quickly on this occasion. However, on another occasion the patient could have been behind that door, in extremis, and very grateful for Tim's earth-shattering arrival!

And the Ugly!

It was dusk on a Friday, and a call came in from a diabetic lady living alone nearby, saying that she was hypoglycaemic, and could I come before she loses consciousness.

After offering advice, I was quick on the draw and out in my car to the house, knowing where she lived. It was getting dark, and I roared into the dark gravel drive. I could see there was a light on behind the side door.

No response from ringing the bell.

'Hello,' I called.

Not a sound, not a murmur.

I ventured into the hall, opening and closing doors, looking into rooms, searching for the patient in the large rambling house.

I entered a dimly lit lounge, and that's when my heart skipped a beat. Now, I like dogs and I'm not normally scared of them, but Staffies are a breed apart, a force of nature. There, on the far side of the room, was a white bundle of muscle, short powerful legs, small pink eyes and a huge salivating jaw ready to deal with the lanky stranger who had made the mistake of entering into its space. As our eyes locked, it didn't bark but growled and made its move towards me. They call it fight or flight, and fortunately flight made the right call. Somehow, I managed to reverse out of the door and shut it just as the dog was airborne. An Exocet. Bang! The door boomed as the dog hit the door like a cannonball. Alarmingly, silence followed; however, I was not going to wait around to undertake a Glasgow coma score on the Staffie, and so I shot upstairs, checking more doors for the hypoglycaemic patient. I eventually found the lady in a spare bedroom, barely conscious, lying recumbent on the bed. Glucose was quickly administered intravenously, and as the patient became more lucid, she enquired,

'I hope Bertha did not give you any problems. She is not good with strangers.'

Not good with strangers! Now that is what I call an understatement!

'No, no problems at all,' I mumbled, not wanting to reveal my agitated state to myself or to the patient, at this juncture.

On the way out, I could hear rustling behind the lounge door so assumed Bertha was now fine and dandy, and

I exited the property quickly. I often wonder, however, what would have happened if I had ventured further into that room before realising the error of my ways. I dread to think what the consequences would have been for my legs and also the diabetic patient. This truly was thinking on my feet!!

Common themes in these three scenarios are impaired communication, due to patient absence or incapacity, alongside a desire for patient safety. Decision-making was swift, pragmatic and courageous/ foolhardy, depending on your viewpoint. At the start of this essay, I asked the reader to consider what happens when communication misfires: results that vary from the good, to the bad and to the ugly!

23

THE SHOW MUST GO ON!

2012

'Andrew, Dad's died, what do I do?'

This was my sister speaking to me on the phone in my consulting room one Saturday morning, during surgery. A sledgehammer to the psyche, a punch in the guts.

The problem was, I had a young woman sitting in front of me with acute asthma, and I was on my own at the surgery.

'What happened?' I enquired of my sister Susan.

'He didn't answer my regular morning call, so I came round to check and found him slumped in his chair. I think he was just getting up, putting his boots on and just died peacefully.' Poor Dad, poor Susan. Tears welled.

This was all too much. I needed time to process the information. 'Susan, can you give me a minute, and I'll ring you back, as I need to sort something out.'

Putting the phone down, I turned to the asthmatic patient and said, 'Let's carry on.'

It was evident that the young woman was struggling and had had a very disturbed night. Her peak flow was significantly down, and she was obviously distressed.

'Come through next door, and we will give you some nebulised Ventolin and see if that helps,' I explained, taking her to my side room where the oxygen and salbutamol were kept. I attached the mask and informed her that I would keep popping in.

I quickly needed to get back to my sister, who was hanging on, and in view of the fact that my father had died suddenly and unexpectedly, I suggested that she get the emergency services. She was a brick and duly proceeded through the processes associated with sudden death.

I was a wreck, but back to the patient on the nebuliser. She was slightly less distressed, and her peak flow had come up somewhat, but I was not happy to let her depart just yet with home treatment; in truth, I didn't know what to do. I could not think. I was in turmoil.

Some hospital admissions are barn door; it is obvious when a patient needs to go into hospital. Some are more subtle, and a legion of indicators, some overt and some covert, lead to a decision to admit that on occasions can be intuitive. I had had a patient in her 50s with very subtle symptoms, no signs and no more than a flavour of a problem. I referred her to the emergency stroke unit where an MRI revealed a right-sided cerebral infarct. If quizzed, it was maybe only one or two subtle points in her history, striking a chord, that led me in this direction. One of my mantras was, 'If your waters are telling you to admit, then admit.'

The problem on this occasion was I just couldn't think clearly. I was juggling the management of acute asthma with the death of my father, back and forth in a mental frenzy. I had to play it safe, however, and if this young patient was admitted unnecessarily then so be it. I discussed the admission with the patient, and she was happy to go into hospital for a few hours or for a night at most. It was not my most erudite case description to the hospital admission sister, but it would have to do; I was playing safe. I now needed to get back to my sister quickly, to check how she was doing and then get on with the rest of the Saturday surgery patients, who were by now queuing up.

It is amazing the restorative effects of a cup of tea in troubled times, and so before carrying on with the surgery, I sat down and took stock for five minutes with a cup in my hand. My mind wandered between my sister, informing Annie and the children of their grandfather's death, and memories of my parents.

My mother had died suddenly twelve years previously of a pulmonary embolus, after surgery for colorectal cancer. This came as a real shock, and what I am still not able to process is that I did not talk to her enough about how she was feeling and express my love for her before she died. Her unexpected death still lives with me today, and why is this? Communication. I was not going to make the same mistake twice, and so as my father struggled on without mum, I made a point of talking to him on an emotional level, discussing everything with him from sex through to the state of the nation. This was fine, but the most important message of all to convey, however, was how much we treasured him as a family.

I had known my father could not go on for ever, as he was by this time eighty-four. I had spoken to his cardiothoracic surgeon after his bypass operation and knew his coronary arteries were pretty shot. Despite this, he had made the most of his life, with plenty of active and interesting pursuits, aided and abetted by my brother and sister, who lived locally to him. Two days before his death, he had delivered a long and detailed lecture on evolution to a local history group, so when his departure came, it still came as a massive shock, and I was very grateful to my siblings for dealing with his sudden death and financial affairs so ably.

My sister still feels guilty about disturbing me in the surgery to this day. She shouldn't, as she was the one on the ground having to deal with the trauma of our father's death. She was the one who phoned him every day and made sure that he was coping on a weekly basis. I feel indebted to her. On that particular Saturday morning, I just had to keep going and continue seeing my patients: the show must go on. This is just how the system worked in years gone by, with more latitude given nowadays to personal circumstances. Where the correct balance lies on the scale between dealing with the patient and one's personal life is open to continuing debate in medical circles under the idiom 'work–life balance.' On that morning, however, I am pretty sure that my decision to keep going was probably not in the best interests of the asthmatic patient or myself. The problem was, who else was there to do the job? Even when your father dies, it is ever thus.

24

A WINTER'S TALE

2013

Half time at Ipswich Town Football Club, and Town were beating Derby, with the scoreline reflected in the positive atmosphere of the crowd. The bar area below the Bobby Robson Lower Stand was as raucous as ever, with the beer and pies flying out at a rate of knots. I was talking to Tom and enquired about his mum, Teresa, who had been our practice nurse practitioner for over thirty years.

'She is the most professional person I have ever met. I work with hundreds of people in London, and none of them can hold a candle to my mum,' stated Tom firmly, making me wonder why he was saying this here and now and with such conviction. What point was he trying to make?

Sad person that I am, I returned to the conversation in my mind a few days later and delved into the notions and definitions of professionalism and what being a professional really means. There is obviously something about being a member of a profession, but more importantly being a professional person includes being competent and skilful, and exhibiting a courteous, conscientious and business-like manner in the workplace. This is how Tom felt about his mum, and I was left thinking that he was absolutely correct to use the term professional in relation to her. There is, however, one trait that is not quite included above, and that is dedication. What is this trait where people go over and above any standard job remit or role to provide a service? Well, this is a short story from our neck of the woods concerning Teresa. It goes some way in explaining what dedication to the patient and to work is all about.

It was winter in Botesdale, and heavy snowfall was expected during the night. As the health centre staff were leaving at the end of the day, I heard various people voice their concerns about getting to work the next day. Teresa piped up,

'I have got a lot of patients coming in tomorrow, so if the snow is really bad, I will have to walk.'

This was despite living over 4 miles away and being 20 weeks' pregnant with baby Anna! I was busy doing paperwork, but this statement must have entered into my subconscious because the next morning as everyone trooped in, kicking snow off their boots, with no sign of Teresa, I thought 'Oh no, she's walking! She is going to walk from Blo' Norton.'

The village is known for its high winds, which maybe explained the Blo part.

Following a quick conflab with a few others, I rang Grant, Teresa's husband.

'Grant, is Teresa with you?'

'No, she is walking to work. I couldn't stop her. She was up and off at the crack. We are completely snowed in here with all the roads closed.'

'It's seriously cold out there, Grant. Shall I drive towards you as far as I can and see if she is on her way? Is she on the roads or going over the fields?'

'The roads. Would you mind, Andy, as I am really worried about her?' His anxiety barrelled down the line.

So, I was off out into the snow in my trusty red VW Polo to look for our practice nurse, who had quite literally gone off piste. I drove slowly for about a mile, half way through the village of Redgrave, and there I saw a solitary figure coming up the hill looking in good fettle but slightly tired around the gills.

'Are you alright, Teresa? Do you want a lift?'

'OK, thanks, but I'm OK really.'

After some thought, Teresa got in the car; however, despite the respite from the cold, I could tell she was a little put out at being helped and taxied to the surgery. Because of this, I informed her that I had had a word with Grant, who was worried and was now waiting to hear what had happened.

As the morning wore on with everyone on track and the surgeries on time, some bright spark ventured,

'How is she going to get back home?' Oh great, another problem!

Fortunately, a wonderful Norfolk shepherd, Brian, was in the surgery that morning and had arrived in his tractor to guarantee safe arrival for his appointment. We collared him.

'Brian, can you wait around a while and give Teresa a lift back to her place at the end of the morning? Would you mind staying here until then?'

Brian was a brick. 'No problem. A pleasure, Doctor.'

'Please use our staff lounge, and help yourself to tea and coffee, while you wait.'

At the allotted hour, Brian and Teresa had an adventurous return, with the cab of the tractor offering some comfort from the cold and providing a panoramic view of the snow-clad journey back to Blo' Norton.

We did not discuss this incident until recently, when I was considering writing these stories, and I enquired why she was slightly perturbed about being driven the final part of the journey.

'It was because by walking to work I was making it quite clear that being pregnant during a heavy snowfall was not going to get in the way of my work. When women take time off during pregnancy, it can be cast in a negative light, and I did not want that to happen to me. Who was going to see the patients, anyway? It also happened to be one of the most beautiful and memorable walks I have ever undertaken.'

'Which I then interrupted,' I replied, feeling slightly guilty.

'No, don't worry; it was getting a bit much, and it was nice to get to the end quickly.'

So, what does it take to be seen as dedicated as well as professional in this day and age when these values appear to be eroded by targets, inspection teams and adverse media coverage? Well, I would venture that being considered courteous, competent and conscientious was not enough for Teresa in this case, making her prepared to walk to work under the most trying of circumstances! Whether this was entirely wise, I am not so sure; however, she was prepared to take a calculated risk in getting to work to see her patients that morning. Such acts of dedication occur a thousand times a day in the NHS, and I have been lucky enough to witness some of them along the way. Normally occurring in health facilities and hospitals the length and breadth of the country, only a handful, however, involve a shepherd, a tractor and lashings of snow!

25

THE RULE OF THREES

2013

My grannie was a wise old owl. Stashed away in her pantry was a pile of old crockery. After two slices of bad luck, she would smash one of these plates in order to pre-empt the third bit of misfortune. Not normally superstitious, Grannie was no fool; she knew a thing or two about life. You never know, if I had followed suit, I may have avoided a ghastly trip to an Italian hospital with Annie, which still haunts me to this day. So buckle up and brace yourself, as we have a fair way to go with this tale.

It was winter, South Tyrol, and we were doing what? You got it, skiing. I know, I know, you will say we were asking for trouble, but we had enjoyed a disaster-free decade of downhill. Our party on this occasion was not the usual group of seasoned skiers but a cheerful group of friends and family of mixed ability who had come along for the ride. Good snow, clear skies, nice company. What could go wrong in our short four-day trip, hey? Plenty!

Day one. Booted and suited, we were high up on the slopes, a large party scattered across the hill in small groups and making our way down the relatively straightforward pistes of Ladurnes, a small resort south of Innsbruck. Now, strange as it may sound, although Annie and I embrace skiing with its unique sense of freedom, exhilaration and expression, what we really enjoy is the blue sky, mountain air and coffee in the cosy alpine chalet huts. One hut in particular was our favourite: Ladurnerhutte, owned by an old friend, Martin Keim, with coffee and strudel to die for. No sooner had we been greeted by Martin with the cheerful, 'The English family has arrived,' and sat down with our coffee, our friend Gary appeared looking concerned.

'Dawn has been hit by a snowboarder and can't remember what happened. We are concerned she may have been knocked out cold.'

A head injury with retrograde amnesia did not sound good to me, and so in a blur of activity we managed to get Dawn down the mountain and into an ambulance on her way to the local hospital in Vipiteno for a check. Now, for some reason, which must have centred on a sense of professional duty, I elected to stay with Dawn and go with her to the hospital, leaving her brother Gary to organise everyone else. To this day, I have this probably misplaced moral obligation to bundle into situations where I feel I can offer medical help. So, five minutes later, I was hurtling to the hospital sandwiched between ambulance staff at the front, with Dawn stretchered out in the back. Slightly shell shocked, I realised the error of my ways when there was a tap on my shoulder and a clipboard carefully passed to me with the following request in broken English.

'Scusi, your wife's details on the form, please.'

I had a slight problem with this one, as since I had last seen Dawn many years ago, she had got married, changed job and moved. Seeing that the form required name, date of birth and address, even the basics alluded me. I had to hand the pen and clipboard back, meekly mumbling with a Gallic shrug,

'She is not my wife! Sorry.'

With an expression flitting across the face of the paramedic in the back that registered 'who is this joker,' the form was duly retracted. I carried on in silent reverie, thinking, 'Oh my God, I am deep into the solids here. They think I am Dawn's husband, and I don't even know who she is. I am not even sure she is really called Dawn. All I know for sure is that she's Gary's sister, at least I hope she is!'

During the course of the morning in hospital, I would be called through to be with Dawn with the forbidding and slightly Teutonic command, 'Dawn's husband, please,' at which point I would trudge through to see Dawn looking ever more alert and with it, having suffered only a mild case of concussion. A measure of her recovery was the increasing look of embarrassment written across her face when I blundered into her room and sat by the bedside. Rather than real husband Nick or brother Gary, she was essentially confronted by a total stranger looking down at her partially disrobed supine state. Eventually, enough was enough, and in view of the likelihood of discharge that day, I contacted brother Gary to come and relieve the situation before we encountered more sham marital embarrassment. To this day, Dawn introduces me as her second husband by proxy, as I am glad to say she survived the first day of our holiday debacle.

Day two, and our party had enjoyed a fulsome session skiing, still in one piece. The hotel had arranged an evening game of curling on the ice rink opposite, for those intrepid enough to brave the cold, whilst the remaining faint-hearted souls retired back to the warmth of the hotel bar or bed. So it was no surprise to those folk who know me that I took option two and could be found reclining in my room relaxing. Half asleep, I heard running on the stairs, followed by shouting from daughter Hannie on the landing.

'Dad, dad!' The bedroom door burst open.

'Dad, a guy has slipped over on the rink, hit his head and has blood running out of his ear. I have been sent to get you. You've got to come now!'

'Blood out of his ear, Hannie. Are you sure?'

'Yes, Dad. Stop asking questions. You have got to come now. Move it.'

With that she was gone, whilst I bumbled around looking for my boots and jacket and then headed out across the road and onto the rink. My God it was treacherous in boots at that time of night.

Sure enough, lying on the ice shrouded in blankets, was one of the other hotel guests, Paul from Yorkshire, eyes open, able to speak quite coherently, and a large pool of blood on the ice creeping from his right ear. I initially hoped that he had lacerated his scalp; however, closer inspection revealed that the blood was definitely discharging from the ear canal and meant only one thing. The slip on the ice, and resultant fall on the back of the head, had fractured this poor chap's skull base. This was serious stuff, and fortunately an ambulance had been called. My only options were to keep him warm, head still and neck supported. In a matter of a few minutes, I heard the shrill alarm of an Italian Job ambulanza, followed by the opening of heavy doors and the clomp, clomp of paramedic boots on ice. Clomp, clomp reverberating through the ice, getting closer and then for a split second, nothing. A whoomf and a grunt. I looked around, and to my disbelief there was the paramedic lying on his back like a beetle, having also gone over on the ice, his fall broken by a large rucksack. Lucky for him, bad for the medical equipment in the rucksack. Undeterred, the paramedic was up and over like a flash, and using a scoop stretcher we carefully got Paul into the ambulance, and he was off.

Paul, accompanied by his steadfast wife, faced a long journey to a neurological centre south of Bolzano, where he remained an inpatient for a couple of weeks. Fortunately, I can report that the bleeding stopped relatively quickly, and Paul made a good recovery and is back skiing again. That is a Yorkshireman for you! Two accidents in two days requiring hospital admission, so during dinner that evening nerves were jangling within the party.

Day three, and boy do I regret not taking one of my grannie's plates on holiday! A well-worn skiing maxim is that accidents often happen on the last ski run of the day. Fatigue, poor light, slush, moguls or ice can all increase the likelihood of an accident. So it was with this in mind that we all diligently packed up our skis and returned them to the ski hire shop. Then someone in our party fancied a final run on a toboggan after a restorative cup of coffee. Bad move, as I should have clocked that the last ski run of the day can also apply to last toboggan run. Before we knew it, most of our party were halfway up the mountain sitting on toboggans ready to slide down the mountain to the car park at the bottom. Five kilometres of fun, hey? I took off and found I was going faster than expected, and on careering round a corner, I saw a couple of members of our party standing to the side of the track. Shooting past, I got to the bottom, with a feeling of dread. Where is Annie? She took off before me. No sign. I started to walk back up the track on the edge of the run, before I saw her coming down in some pain.

Looking pale, she explained,

'I was going quite fast and came across someone standing on the path. I was worried I may injure them, so I veered off and crashed into the wooden barrier. The impact jarred my back, threw me up in the air, and I landed on my coccyx. My back and coccyx really hurt.'

Now, Annie has a high pain threshold, and if she says she is in pain, I am writhing in agony. This long experience has taught me to take her symptoms more than seriously, and so with an intuitive dread, I knew she had suffered a fractured thoracic vertebrae and needed to go to the hospital. Annie, however, wanted to get back to the hotel, have a hot bath and see how things go. I will never forget helping her to get undressed and into the bath. Damp shoes and socks carefully removed, salopettes unclipped and unzipped. A gentle lowering of her normally robust but now fragile body into the hot water. I was fighting back the tears. Both of us were hoping for pain relief, but sadly there was none to be had. It was the hospital we needed. Again. Our third brush with the Italian health service in three long days.

As we were a walk-in casualty, the hospital was sceptical as to the extent of the injuries; however, once the Xrays returned indicating two thoracic fractures and a split coccyx, they stepped up. We were due to fly home the next day, and without Annie's courage and a hefty dose of OxyContin, I am not sure we would have made it back. Make it home we did, and after three months of rest and recuperation Annie made a good recovery. The nightmare was over.

I still feel slightly nauseated when thinking about this short trip to the Tyrol, with emotions that vary from anxiety through to guilt and anger. What did we learn? Well, when taking to the slopes with newcomers of mixed abilities, take things carefully. Beware of ice, as even when you know it is hazardous, the reality of falling over is at least painful and at times deadly; curling rinks are no exception! Do not be tempted to have a final go at anything, and I mean anything, that involves hurtling yourself downhill late on in the day. Finally, and critically, be prepared to smash something after the second accident because the rule of three will find you out!

26

THE END OF THE BEGINNING
OR THE BEGINNING OF THE END?

'A RETIREMENT STREAM OF CONSCIOUSNESS'
2016

I am sitting in a conference room of the De Vere West One Hotel, Portland Place, London, gazing out at the art deco façade of the BBC building. Nostalgia stirs as the autumnal sunshine falls on the limestone walls, awakening memories of my medical student days in nearby Charlotte Street.

Keep with it, Andrew, you are due to give a lecture in a few minutes on achieving the recently introduced 28 Day to Diagnosis Cancer Targets to a large hostile audience of clinicians and hospital managers. This is not a time for reminiscence, as a previous speaker is getting a rough ride during question time. Someone is asserting that the patriarchal stance taken by many GPs in cancer communication is unacceptable. No doubt true, sometimes, but not now please, as I am the only GP on the bill today. I see a grilling coming with this lot, and so keep up, Andrew. Please, keep up.

Here we go again, it is that damned autumnal light awakening my memory again. I am across the road outside the BBC during my first freshers' week, trying to persuade Radio 1 DJ Simon Bates to come back to the medical school bar on his way home, where there is one hell of a party kicking off. This is Treasure Hunt Night, when we were given licence to accrue a series of items to adorn the bar, including hot dog stands, celebrities, strippers, professors, cars, and everything bar the kitchen sink. Despite ultimately dragging Simon Bates down to the bar, we stood no chance, as the crew who lived in the red-light area of Soho always won The Treasure Hunt hands down with a plethora of adornments, including the aforementioned strippers! For a fleeting second, I bask in the warmth of happy memories.

Oh shit, rouse yourself, Andrew.

'I would now like to introduce Dr Andrew Yager, Macmillan GP from Suffolk. Andrew has a particular interest in the primary and secondary care interface in relevance to cancer care.'

I was up and before I knew it had the projector remote in my hand and was delivering my prepared talk, including a question on patriarchal GPs!

Why am I relaying these mental juxtapositions to you now? Well, despite there being quite a lot of work sandwiched in the middle, I suppose whilst looking out at Portland Place I was thinking about the beginning of my medical life whilst winding the clock down at the back end. I have retired as a partner at Botesdale, have slowly reduced my clinical work in the surgery and I'm now working for Macmillan in a role that hopes to make cancer pathways work as efficiently as possible in Suffolk. This is why I am lucky enough to be sitting in a swanky London hotel in the first place. A role that is in turn interesting, rewarding and has real value in that pathway efficiency relates to cancer survival. Rewarding though the Macmillan work is, there is no doubt, however, that I feel in the twilight of my career as the clinical contact diminishes. Some people can retire overnight and define a new life, whereas others aim for a slow landing and gradually build a future path for themselves. I am in the latter group, and despite having a full life with many different pursuits outside medicine, I'm finding it harder than anticipated. The problem is that clinical medicine and patient relationships, in particular, have gone viral into my being, and I am struggling to find a cure and rid myself of this affliction. I suspect I am not alone, caught between the medical virus and the need to see more of my family and disengage from ever more challenging clinical work as the years go on and medicine becomes ever more complex.

A passage in Caroline Elton's book *Almost Human* is helpful, along with Helen Rose Fuchs Ebaugh discussing her own personal experiences of leaving her role as a Catholic nun in her study *Becoming an Ex: The Process of Role Exit*:

> *Disengagement from old roles is a complex process that involves shifts in reference groups, friendship networks, relationships with former group members, and most importantly shifts in a person's own sense of self-identity. Exiters can*

*feel in mid-air, ungrounded, nowhere. The future
is unknown and they no longer belong to the past.*

In the early years of a medical career, there is a defined structure for many people, from school right through to the first substantive job. Though the career pathway can be arduous, there are frameworks within different medical careers which I probably took for granted. To avoid becoming a retirement *exiter* suspended in mid-air, the challenge is to dismantle the previous career framework, either quickly or slowly, and build a new structure for the future, around one's personal, social, financial, family and health needs.

Understanding this process and proceeding positively and purposefully are important, if a retirement limbo, characterised by personal drift and inertia, is to be avoided. Tales abound of people in all walks of life who flop over the employment finish line and for one reason or another and through no fault of their own end up adrift and caught in an aimless void. I understand all of this, but how do I proceed? Well, throughout life I have used role models as a guide, and so let me introduce some characters who provide some personal inspiration.

Annie and I had spoken to Eric and Sylvia, then a recently retired GP and a health visitor.

'Don't leave your retirements too late you two, if you can avoid it financially. If you do, you may find that you don't have enough gas in the tank to define your future and make the most of things.'

Wise words, echoing Helen Ebaugh's statement, and at the time I thought Sylvia and Eric should know. You see, they both met at art school and on completing their studies decided to change course and enter their respective health professions. Their creative sparks were not extinguished, however, with a life adorned with stunning projects from model boats, to steam engines, to stained glass, to upholstery and house renovation. Retirement was a chance to turn up the afterburner on this creative energy and redefine themselves. What did they turn to? Stained glass, in view of their shared interest and previous experience. Not a casual hobby but a formal commercial endeavour, and so where did they turn to learn the ancient art of stained-glass painting and fusing, for religious and architectural purposes? Sienna in Italy, no less, living in a caravan for a year and learning the tricks of the trade from local artisans, guilds and tutors.

Next they needed a studio, and what did they acquire? Discarded by a local railway museum, they stumbled upon a Norwegian railway carriage, which they subsequently installed on rails in their garden. Perfect for joint creative crafting, with Sylvia at one end, Eric at the other and a multitude of windows fore and aft for the light. What did they produce from this joint commercial venture? Well, magnificent stained-glass panels for church windows, of which there are a multitude in East Anglia. We have one of their creations in our village church, commemorating the Millennium and featuring the Good Lord on a 2 by 10 foot wired panel. It is spellbinding and poignant at once.

There is a sting in the tail to this story, and a lesson too. Sadly, Eric and Sylvia both died of cancer in their mid-70s. Fortunately, for many of us blessed to have witnessed their creative explosion, it is possible to visit many of their local stained-glass windows and remember the loving ingenious couple who certainly 'defined their futures and made the most of things,' in the relatively short time available to them in retirement.

Roz is a daughter of Kent, with a farming lineage going back generations. Dark curly hair, dark eyes, a farmer's rolling gait and strong hands and thick fingers, she was born to work with the land. In her late teens, however, another calling deflected her from this path: medicine. It was during this time that she had the misfortune to share a flat in Royal Oak, London with an old reprobate: me! Surviving this encounter, Roz entered general practice, returning to Kent where she became a well-respected member of the local community near her place of birth.

Retirement beckoned in her early 60s, but, as with myself, medicine had installed itself into her DNA, and she was finding dealing with the clinical wind down and lack of patient contact traumatic. Around this time, her parents passed away, and being the sole heir, Roz inherited the old Kentish farm, lock, stock and barrel. Whilst coping with bereavement and retirement, Roz now had a working farm to manage. Many people would go for the easy life, cash in their chips and sell the farm, but not the old farmer in Roz. Enter husband

Richard, a geographer who realised that the old pit on the farm was part of a long chalk band stretching from Kent to the Champagne area of France. Interesting, especially when combined with south-facing slopes, the correct grape and a hell of a lot of hard graft. Roz and Richard are now in their sixth year of Chartham Wines, with 17,000 bottles of excellent wine produced last year and Taittinger Champagne recently installed as their new neighbours in a bid to mitigate the effects of global warming. Despite the fact that they have potentially hit commercial gold, the part of the job that Roz really appreciates is working in the vineyard shop. Why? That old virus in the DNA is calling again.

'It is just like general practice, Andrew. Meeting and chatting to loads of different people for short periods of time over the counter. I love it!'

The farming GP has found a spiritual home in retirement through courage, purpose and hard work. A role model indeed.

Now, Andrew, get off your arse and follow your old flatmate's lesson. Stop gazing through the window at Portland Place and immersing yourself in student nostalgia. Put your back into this retirement lark. Continue working as long as your finances and abilities will allow; plan the next stage with Annie; progress with purpose; do not dwell in the past, and embrace the future with gusto. While you are at it, take a leaf out of a certain wartime leader's book and make this phase of your life the end of the beginning, rather than the beginning of the end. Get to it!

27

WONDERFUL TONIGHT

2017

Annie and I are standing at the back of the pub, listening to a local band deliver their version of 'Wonderful Tonight' by Eric Clapton. A moving song at the best of times, and this was the best of times. The band was composed mainly of school friends of my son Nick, all by now in their mid-20s and enjoying the expression and energy of live performance. It was the vocalist and drummer, however, who caught the eye. Taking centre stage, neck extended into the mike, and singing whilst drumming, David was doing a good impression of Phil Collins. Phil Collins now that is, shaven head and all, not a young Phil thirty years ago with hair. So what is the background to Dave's presence in a band of twenty-somethings?

A couple of years after starting at Botesdale, I was in the middle of a morning surgery when the next appointment was with a smiling, bright-eyed middle-aged lady from a local village, in for a routine check-up. Wearing a smart pink jacket over a colourful floral dress and flat sensible shoes, Pat proceeded to explain her medical condition quietly and succinctly. Much thought had gone into how best to explain her symptoms and get the best out of the consultation, making my role straightforward. Having summed up our plan for her next visit, Pat then gave me food for thought.

'If you and your wife ever need a bit of childminding in the future, then give me a ring, as I love looking after children.' Now, thousands of statements are made during the course of medical consultations, but Pat's offer really stuck in my mind that day. Looking back, I think that what struck me most was her kind and solid demeanour, coupled with the simplicity and sincerity of the offer. That evening, I informed Annie that I had met Pat in the surgery, and I explained the kind offer of childcare, which we put firmly on the back boiler, as we were not at that stage thinking of starting a family! Annie was continuing in her nursing career locally, and our priorities were those of many newlyweds: enjoying life, work and setting up a home. So back boiler it was, but not so far back that the idea was dismissed or forgotten.

A couple of years later, Annie fell pregnant, and during this time we discussed how to juggle work and childcare, with Pat's name returning to the fore very quickly. Annie contacted Pat, who came and helped her in the house for a while prior to taking over as childminder to our firstborn, Juliet, when Annie returned to work. We are blessed with three lovely children, who I am very proud to say are all good, decent people. Their ever-loving mother can take all of the credit for this achievement, with the caring and patient Nannie Pat holding the fort and allowing Annie to return to work. Juliet, Nick and Hannie all traversed their childhoods and early teenage years under the kind and watchful eye of Nannie Pat.

So where does David the drummer fit into this? Well David is Pat's son and following a decade-long absence from drumming was winkled out of retirement by Nick and his mates. David was well known to our family, as firstly he is a nice bloke and secondly he used to be quite handy with the sticks. Once a drummer, always a drummer! Before the month was out, the kit was rediscovered in the back of an old polytunnel, dusted down, new skins attached, rhythms remembered and rehearsed, and the average age of the band advanced by a decade.

The show must go on, and indeed the show was going on tonight, with crooning Phil Collins in his stride.

So whilst standing in the pub with a smile on my face, and Annie on my arm, I was reflecting on the various bonds and themes that brought this motley crew of an intergenerational band together. Making music and giving enjoyment to a crowd, albeit a small crowd; family bonds without borders, rivalries or competition; shared stories, of nappies, bottles and tantrums; maternal grace and guidance. And the glue, the heartbeat of this amalgam of friends and family in the audience, well, who else, Annie. She was and always is Wonderful Tonight.

28

IT IS ALL A MATTER OF TIME –
A POLEMIC

2017

I ventured into the health centre one day to check that a patient seen the previous week had received an urgent CT scan appointment. Whilst in, I bumped into John, a remarkably energetic GP in his late 60s, who was in the middle of a surgery. I could not help but notice the rictus smile, the clammy sheen and fixed stare of a doctor under stress.

'Can't stop, Andrew. I was doing fine, but then a patient was late, and the following two patients were incredibly complex. I am hours behind. Bye.'

On how many occasions have I heard this refrain over the years? Time pressure.

In my view, time pressure is the single most important problem within UK general practice. Lengthening consultation times to 15 minutes over the next decade should be the fulcrum around which future primary care services are evolved. In reviewing the evidence below, I am grateful to the June 2018 King's Fund publication, *Innovative Models of General Practice*, which includes the sound Cumbrian GP Hugh Reeve as one of its authors.

Irving et al. in 2017 published in the *BMJ* a review of primary care physician consultation times from

67 countries and found that among economically developed countries the UK had the shortest consultation length at 9.2 minutes. Patients in Sweden had the luxury of 22.5 minutes with their GP, and in Australia 15 minutes. But, get this, the authors estimated that at the current rate of change UK consultation length would only reach 15 minutes by 2086! We will have to wait sixty years to get to where the Aussies are now!

It is all very well sounding off and saying what I want, but what do patients want? Well, it was a while ago, but Wensing et al. published in *Social Science & Medicine* in 1998 a review of 19 international research studies and found that the five most important patient priorities for general practice care were: humaneness, competence/accuracy, patient involvement in decisions, time for care, and accessibility.

Now, the NHS has made a commitment to person-centred care; however, having enough time is critical to both patients and clinicians in delivering this goal. Salisbury et al. in 2013 published research in the *British Journal of General Practice* that found that in practice an average consultation included discussion of 2.5 different problems across a wide range of disease areas. This accords with an audit I undertook about five years ago when I looked at consecutive morning surgeries, each with 18 booked patients, and documented the number of discreet problems raised. I was shocked to find that during an average morning between fifty to sixty problems would be landed at my feet from the 18 patients seen.

My record for problems presented in one consultation was with David, who brought in a drawing of a pin man with thirteen problems that he wanted sorting carefully highlighted. Ouch! Some practices try to mitigate such behaviour by restricting patients to one problem per consultation. I have always resisted this, as symptom presentation can be haphazard, the patient has often had to struggle to get in, and further problems are just put off to another day. So, sticking to my guns, David and I valiantly tried to work through his 13 problems, not in the nationally allocated 9.2 minutes but more like 45 minutes, resulting in a posse of delayed and disgruntled patients in the waiting room.

So, to deliver this person-centred care, the average GP has to wade through 2.5 problems within a potential national average of 9.2 minutes. Would we as patients tolerate this when going to see our accountant, solicitor, or counsellor? No is the answer, and yet we do go along with this aberration within general practice, where the stakes can be sky high. This patient tolerance of the consultation length status quo is something I have never quite got to grips with in thirty years of practice.

I remember an old GP mentor, who is sadly no longer with us, explaining that the central point to general practice training was learning how to manage risk in the time available. In other words, how to be a safe GP. I see risk in the consultation as the danger of inflicting something unpleasant or harmful on a patient through one's action or inaction. A couple of years ago, I published a short article in the *British Journal of General Practice* after I had tried to quantify and audit the perceived risk in my consultations. Out of 314 consultations audited, only 10% had no perceived risk at all, whilst the vast majority had a potential overt or covert risk. Practising safely is of extreme importance to GPs, but put them in a situation where this is impossible for significant slabs of the day and they will vote with their feet and leave. A further nail in the coffin of GP recruitment. Phil Hammond, comedian, journalist and 'Medicine Balls' in the satirical magazine *Private Eye*, gave up general practice because he felt his working environment had become intrinsically unsafe. I will repeat Clare Gerada's words mentioned elsewhere in these essays: 'General practice is practically impossible to do well at the moment. The 10-minute consultation is too short and we are expected to do too much.'

I once saw a nurse and a retired gentleman who both complained of slightly swollen legs. Their symptoms and signs were minimal, but during a careful examination I felt there were enough signs to perform screening of their blood and for subsequent referral for ultrasound scans, all of which took time to explain and organise. Both patients were subsequently found to have deep vein thromboses and as such were at significant risk of pulmonary emboli, a life-threatening condition. Managing such subtle symptoms and signs for danger takes time, and attempts to cut corners will result in disaster at some stage along the road.

So, I would assert that if we are to deliver safe person-centred care in the best interests of patients and medical professionals alike, then we should not wait until 2086. We should strive for 15-minute consultations as soon as possible. The June 2018 King's Fund publication mentions other models of care for releasing time for such GP consultations, but in my view the report did not go far enough. The 15-minute consultation should be the fulcrum around which funding and service redesign are levered. I have been harping on about this for a good fifteen years now and wait with exasperation as the RCGP, BMA, NHSE and HEE deliberate on the problems in primary care without consistently considering consultation length. Some light at the end of the tunnel is coming from some GP out of hours services which mandate defined consultation and surgery length in order to recruit GPs into shifts working antisocial hours. In order to be sustainable, any drive to increase consultation length will have to go hand in hand with further ongoing initiatives to manage GP workload; however, there is no time like the present, because it is all a matter of time.

29

WHERE DO I START?

1991–2019

I have hesitated to write about Dr Tim, as after much thought, I really do not know where to start, or for that matter where to finish. So, I ask you to bear with me if this next story meanders somewhat, mirroring the character involved; however, I think it wise we regroup and try and start at the beginning of our long association.

Our previous senior partner, Bill, had retired, and my remaining partners, Rob and Sue, and I were looking to recruit. We decided to do the job properly, advertise nationally with formal interviews and not rely on local word of mouth. Or so we planned, but I had not bargained on a local barn dance to which Annie and I were invited, and I hadn't bargained on Tim. Annie and I had just got our drinks in hand when a cheerful, solid-looking chap wearing John Lennon glasses careered into us at a rate of knots, pint of beer in one hand and a pretty dark-haired woman called Anna on the other arm. We all exchanged apologies for the significant volumes of alcohol that had disgorged onto the floor from all our glasses and started chatting. Nearly two hours later, I was still talking to a cheerful, solid-looking chap wearing John Lennon glasses. Annie and Anna had very sensibly melded into the tumult, leaving Tim and I to undertake what was probably by now an informal job interview. Having set out to be squeaky clean in our approach to human resources and recruitment, chaos was already beginning to reign.

This chequered interview process resulted in the partnership employing a bright, cheerful, local GP with excellent communication and team skills. What I had not bargained on was the degree of laughter he would bring to proceedings, both from his conversation but also from his behaviour. Let me explain. Three weeks after Tim's arrival, I had just opened the back door of the health centre when I heard the growl of a V8 engine rumbling along the lane. Tim had a yellow Rover P6 2000 with a recognisable engine, and I suspected he was roaring along on his way to work. The next thing, his Rover burst into the car park all guns blazing, at which time Tim saw me standing at the back door. I suspect that as he was new to the job his first thought was to acknowledge my presence and wave, and so when the Rover shot past the back door, he wound down the window, smiling with arm aloft in a show of friendship, rather than attend to his speed. Then I saw the grimace as the car left the tarmac and went up onto the wet grass verge. There was a stamp on the brakes before the car tunnelled into the large hedge on the border between our health centre and the school next door. The car had buried itself so far into the hedge that Tim was trapped. Gales of laughter accompanied the extrication process, which was not altogether straightforward or quick! Indeed, this was an induction period with a difference and indicative of the chaos and laughter that could, would and should ensue!

So, over the years, and despite the odd glitch, I got more and more fond of this large, kind, wise doctor whose personality resembled an old leather armchair for many of us in the surgery. This is an expression borrowed from rugby international Paul Ackford, who used it to describe fellow second row Wade Dooley, and it implies being comfortable in an old, trusted friend's company. This metaphor is very apposite in relation to Tim. Not that he was a pushover, and I remember him once describing himself as more akin to a hippo than an old leather armchair; in other words, very happy to potter around on the bottom of the river bed minding his own business, but when there was trouble on the riverbank he was more than capable of roaring up out of the water with a rare and frightening ferocity. This was an analogy I took seriously, as my uncle, a zoologist at Cambridge University, described the hippo as the most dangerous animal in the bush apart from homo sapiens. To illustrate this, he regaled me with the story of a hippo attacking his Land Rover whilst in Uganda; it fortunately chose the car door rather than himself, removing it at a stroke before trundling off into the bush, the prize door locked between its huge jaws. Talking of car doors . . . Mid-morning on a Tuesday and following the sad death of a very popular village resident, a funeral was about to start in the local church. A call came in that Glenda, on her way to the funeral, had fallen and could the doctor come quickly. Tim was on his way just ahead of the multitude of cars streaming down to the village for the funeral. House found, handbrake on, ignition off, seat belt unbuckled, he reached for the medical bag on the back seat and open the door. Bang and crunch! The car door was now apparently somehow in the road, with the bumper and radiator of one of the fellow mourners not looking too sharp either. OK, Tim was missing a car door, but this was small beer, as an altercation flared, followed by an explanation and an exchange of details, not to mention the stream of cars behind waiting in line patiently and the delay the accident had caused to the start of the funeral. Just as the hippo in my uncle's tale had taken off with a door, Tim now did the same with equal aplomb. We have all done such things, just some of us have done them more often than others!

On a serious note, though I worked with Tim for thirty years, there was always one aspect of his work that eluded me: his consultation technique. During the 1990s, consultation skills training became a big deal in general practice, spearheaded by Jonathan Silverman and Julie Draper, who worked close by in Cambridge. We were encouraged to weave the patient's agenda and medical agenda together simultaneously to great effect. Their subsequent worldwide publications made quite an impact on those of us who had proceeded through medical school with precious little training in such skills. As a teaching practice, this new development heralded a significant amount of in-house consultation skills training; however, Tim never really saw the need to engage with it all. He did not see further training as necessary, as his consultation technique was entirely intuitive, truly unique and very effective indeed. He would naturally weave together the patient and medical agendas when needed, but this process frequently played second fiddle to the patient's social and personal history. Patients would come and see me and say they had been to see Dr Cooke and had become distracted by a long talk on woodcarving or gardening, for instance, not sure they had told him what their problem was. On the contrary, I cannot remember a time when he had missed a diagnosis, did not attend to a patient's agenda or had a substandard entry in the notes: a model GP! It was all just done off the cuff, his acute awareness of the patient's psychology and social history allied to an extremely bright mind stuffed with medical and general knowledge. Being more formulaic about my consultation structure, I still do not understand how it was possible to have such in-depth conversations about social interests within the limited time frame of UK general practice consultations. The art of general practice at its most sophisticated is like watching a skilled conjuror; I am still baffled by this sleight of hand to this day!

So we are now both nearing the end of our respective careers in general practice. Two idiosyncratic working colleagues who became buddies, who became older and possibly wiser and are now about to bow out together. There was more than the occasional cross word but no long-lasting resentment or rancour, just humour and a common bond in our work. Despite my retiring as a partner first, I remained working in the health centre and helping out when the situation demanded. When my old mucker retired, it was time to say au revoir to my

GP life and the magic of Botesdale Health Centre once and for all. It was a long journey of thirty-five years, mostly enjoyable but at times arduous, and no doubt it was made all the more colourful and viable by the solid-looking chap with the John Lennon glasses!

30

MISSION IMPOSSIBLE, OR IS IT?

2017

'The mystery of human existence lies not in just staying alive, but in finding something to live for.'
Fyodor Dostoyevsky, The Brothers Karamazov.

The weft and warp of human personality has always interested me. Never more so than when presented with a person who remains motivated and purposeful, especially when the chips are down. From my meagre experience in general practice, this trait appears in all ages, genders and walks of life, discerned by a bearing, a look in the eye, a timbre to the voice and a story to tell. This is all very fine and dandy when life has a way to course, but what about those individuals who know they are coming to the end of the road and still have a burning mission aflame in their hearts? How do these remarkable individuals manage the mental juxtaposition of limited time and achievement, knowing that it is unlikely they will live to see the fruits of their labours? Being a pessimist and prone to a hysterical mental paralysis when confronted with life-defining symptoms within myself, the answer is I have no idea how it is done. Maybe this explains the source of my own fascination in this personality type. However, I am willing to learn and would like to introduce two characters who have shown me a thing or two. Bob and David.

Strangers to each other, these two men shared the same sense of desire. Both were in their sixties when I knew them and had a long-term cancer diagnosis significantly affecting longevity. They both had a love of cricket, strong and resourceful families, and a very large dose of purpose in their lives.

I got to know Bob several years ago, as he ran the local cancer patient group at the hospital in Bury St Edmunds. He came across as a friendly and wise voice within the small group of patients who gave up their time to improve the running of the NHS cancer services. Quiet for most of the time, Bob would only speak up when he had something of value to say, and when Bob spoke, people listened. It was his voice that I found engaging, in that there was a youthfully eager tone to the delivery with just a slight catch of a serious underlying debility incurred during months of chemotherapy and a bone marrow transplant for lymphoma. Bob knew his health status and longevity were severely compromised, but despite this he had reasons for living, which included using his skills in industry to try and improve local cancer services. Bob needed to influence these meetings and events, getting his point across and driving change whilst somehow casting aside the day-to-day struggles that follow serious illness.

Now, I came under Bob's radar as he had an interest in improving cancer services within primary care and ensuring hospital and general practice worked in synch together for the benefit of the patient. So, one afternoon, following a particularly stuffy meeting, Bob ambles over to me and takes the wind out of my sails with his next question.

'Are you a cricket fan, Andrew?'

'England v India, Edgbaston. Only one cricket match to my name, I am afraid, Bob. Great fun though.'

'How do you fancy coming down to Lords in a couple of months' time, to watch Middlesex versus Yorkshire? I am a member of Middlesex County Cricket Club, you see, and get tickets for guests. I would like to invite you along. It should be a good day out. We can watch cricket as well as discuss my plans for ensuring cancer patients get a good deal from primary care.'

I weigh up the option of working versus visiting the holy grail of cricket. An easy one this!

'That would be great, Bob. Thank you very much.'

The walk from the underground on a hot July day in St John's Wood, London, was glorious, albeit slightly tiring. Standing outside the main entrance to Lord's, I waited for Bob, who had shunned a taxi and undertaken the walk as well. Looking drained, he ushered me into the ground and then introduced me to his initial priorities – a drink, some food, cricket, and then another drink. The term, 'making the most of,' came to mind.

During the day, we roamed the Pavilion, admiring the Long Room, Roof Terrace and portraits of famous cricketers. I wanted to bottle the experience. My consciousness was dimming as Bob's desire to show me a good time included introducing me to the full array of bars in the ground. By the time play was concluded with a Middlesex win, Bob and I were undoubtedly worse for wear. A taxi was deemed necessary for our return to Liverpool Street Station, and we departed happy men, or so I thought initially. Waving each other goodbye at the station, I was aware that there was something missing, which I could not put my finger on at first. Sobering up on the train home, I realised that we had not spent enough time talking about Bob's plans for cancer patients in primary care, and when we did discuss the matter, I had been slightly evasive as I was not sure we could deliver his vision. I was concerned I had slightly let him down. At our next meeting, I endeavoured to correct this omission with Bob, and, indeed, on raising the issue of cancer care for patients in general practice, his focus returned and the ember reignited.

You see, enjoying life to the full is important, but what also counted for Bob on that day with me was the desire to see his vision transformed into local policy in the time left to him. The man had a purpose, carrying him forward through adversity. A benign mission, for a gentle man, but a mission no less. I am pleased to say that his wish is being delivered, as we now have support for Suffolk cancer patients throughout their cancer journey, from hospital care into general practice. Sadly, however, Bob is no longer with us, as he passed away peacefully two years after our trip to Lord's. His legacy lives on, as does my memory for his love of life, his family and Lord's cricket.

Earlier on, I described David as having shared many of the same attributes as Bob. A love of cricket, strong family, serious illness and a burning sense of purpose. I knew David for nearly as long as I have known Annie – he is my brother-in-law, married to Annie's sister, Moira. An architect by trade, David had the ability to see the constructed environment in alternative ways to most people; visionary at times and jarring at others. An abiding memory is of David sitting on the steps of the Place Georges, Pompidou, simply staring at the Pompidou Centre itself, an intense, fixated half smile on his face, legs folded and back hunched. The ground-breaking inside–outside nature of the Rogers and Piano building encapsulated David's own way of seeing design, with the norm replaced by daring and imagination. An optimistic sense of hope for our immediate human habitat infused his being, to the point of borderline delusion. As an architect, it was not a bad place to start, even if the end point could occasionally clash with the status quo and authority.

Sadly, several years ago, David was diagnosed with renal cell carcinoma, and following a decade of life-prolonging but debilitating treatment, the cancer spread to his lungs and bones. Instead of admitting defeat, his imagination went on a flight of fancy, giving him the desire to keep looking forward whilst embracing an attenuated life. Despite his difficult circumstances, his mind was elsewhere, focussed on the problems occurring down the road from his home, at nearby Heathrow Airport, where flight congestion, pollution, and concerns around a third runway are constant. Reconfiguring flight services from the capital involved devising a bold plan for a future 'London Airport.' Despite a bleak future, David's body and being were sustained not only by his remarkable family but also by the hope and mission contained within his imaginative airport plan, for months if not years through to the penultimate day of his life. A bleak prognosis one day from a consultant on the hospital ward was somehow enough to disturb his equanimity, and the following day David died peacefully. The reality of David's circumstance crashed into his hitherto impregnable mental construct, resulting in an overnight downturn in his physical state. Despite the change in his condition resulting in a terminal state, what were David's final words to son Henry?

'Don't forget Airport London.'

You see, David was determined to pass on the burning torch within. Right to the end, he did not give up on his vision.

At the start of this essay, I said I was willing to learn from David and Bob and understand how they kept going despite the difficulties of dealing with long-term illnesses. Well, what I think they both had in common was a quiet optimism, bucket loads of courage and a purpose to get hold of and face the day. In Dostoyevsky's words, they had something to live for, using their sense of mission and imagination to improve life around them. Nowadays, more and more cancer patients are having ongoing treatment for cancer and surviving but finding themselves not fully cured. The social and psychological outfall from this living with cancer is immense, requiring ongoing support and help. This ongoing need for help is now being increasingly recognised throughout the Health Service and third-sector charities such as Macmillan, as not everyone has the resources held by the remarkable Bob and David.

31

CUM SCIENTIA CARITAS

2018

Cum Scientia Caritas, the motto of the Royal College of General Practitioners, means compassion with knowledge. There is a clear resonance within this phrase in relation to working as a doctor, and especially as a GP. Indeed, when prospective medical students come and discuss their future career choice, they frequently advance that they are drawn to medicine because the discipline combines science with concern for people. Medicine works when the compassion and the science are in harmony. You cannot have the one without the other. Prospective medical students appear to understand this relationship intuitively; however, at times in our medical careers, it is possible to lose balance and find oneself pulled to one side or the other. Let me try and explain with a couple of examples from each side of the coin.

I attended an oncology conference in Brighton in 2019. International speakers and nine hundred delegates were packed into one of the huge seafront hotels. All costs were sponsored by Big Pharma. It was big business meets big medicine, with hordes of young doctors strutting their stuff. Punchy.

Before the conference, I had dutifully selected which side lectures and discussions to attend, covering different areas of oncological interest, including colorectal and lung cancer. Normally, I am not prone to social anxiety; however, when blundering into these sessions, I was confronted with academics and medics from all parts of the globe presenting research papers on treatments that seemed rarefied and at times extreme to say the least. My medical day-to-day was poles apart from the other delegates in the room. I felt quashed, concerned for the average patient, and interested as to whether others felt the same. This was medical science in its pure, pioneering, triumphant form; macho medicine on the march, with the patient as a person coming a distant second. Where was the tender holism in all of this, the kindness and the compassion? Wandering along the lush carpets of the hotel corridors, I felt a stranger in my own profession, edgy and introverted. Medicine as pure medical science without relevance to the whole person seemed to strip away the role of the job in relation to humankind. I was witnessing one extreme end of the equation and did not like what I saw. To examine the other side, I need to take you back about twenty years to an event which I hope has relevance.

'This is Mrs Smith, is that the doctor?'

'Yes, Dr Yager speaking.'

'My husband has taken a turn for the worse. Can you come quickly, Doctor?'

I looked at my watch, the hands at 1.30am. This could take a while, I thought, but, still, I should be in the warm soon enough.

'Alright, I will be along now.'

Mr Smith had advanced cancer, and our practice had been looking after his palliative care for some time. I had been along to see him earlier the previous day and so knew the particulars of the case. I knew that Mrs Smith would not ask for a visit in the middle of the night without serious concerns. With that, I was up and off, out of the village and on to the winding lanes.

I knocked on the door of the picture-perfect cottage on the outskirts of a neighbouring village.

The small door was opened by an even smaller occupant, Mrs Smith, dressed in floral apron and frock, sleeves rolled up ready for action.

'Thank you for coming quickly, Doctor. I think he might have passed away.'

'Are you sure?'

'Yes, he just slipped away, just as I came up from the kitchen. I was next to him when he went. He is upstairs.'

I followed Mrs Smith up the winding, narrow staircase and stumbled onto the landing and into the cosy front bedroom. Under the orange glow of the bedside lights, there was Mr Smith lying peacefully on the bed in his pyjamas, obviously dead. The shipshape room was an oasis of calm and comfort, and quickly I confirmed that he was dead and turned to Mrs Smith.

'You are right, he has passed away. I am very glad it was peaceful and you were with him, Mrs Smith. You did a very good job of caring for him.'

'Thank you.'

'Had you thought about calling an undertaker?'

'No, not yet, as I was waiting for you to come.'

'When you are ready, maybe give them a call.'

'I will, but first I want to give him a wash and get him ready for leaving the house. I was wondering if you would help me wash him, Doctor?'

It was then that I noticed the formal suit hanging up on the door of the wardrobe, the rolled-up sleeves on Mrs Smith's forearms, the bowl of water with soap and flannel. I realised that this was no casual request and saw my smart return to bed disappearing into the dawn. I could make an excuse and leave this to the undertakers; however, there was a softly spoken earnestness to Mrs Smith's request that brooked no dissent. I could not say no, and before I could stop myself, I answered, 'Alright, I can stay and help if you would like.'

'Thank you, Doctor.'

The next hour was spent helping Mrs Smith with her ministrations as she slowly and lovingly ensured that Mr Smith looked as smart as possible for his final voyage out of the house. This was not part of any religious practice as far as I was aware but an expression of love for her husband. I suspect Mrs Smith looked after Mr Smith's attire all their married life, and in death he was certainly not going to leave looking scruffy! Helping her turn and lift him while she carefully tended to him was curiously mesmerising and deeply touching. In a positive, practical way, Mrs Smith was coming to terms with her husband's death. Eventually, with a pat on Mr Smith's chest, she declared that she was finished, happy with his looks.

I then took my leave while she waited for the undertaker. 'Thank you once again, Doctor.'

Now, I have included this story as I wanted to explore my motivation for staying behind and helping. Was it professionally driven, an example of kindness or compassion, or a little slice of both? Certainly, no clinical knowledge was involved – far from it. The professional guidance of the General Medical Council talks of being considerate; however, compassion and kindness seem to go that little bit further down the line: they are easy to lose sight of in the hurly-burly of the clinical world, but they affirm our humaneness both to our patients as well as to ourselves as doctors. Quoting from lawyer Kenneth Schwartz in his article for the *Boston Globe* magazine in 1995 following his admission to the Massachusetts General Hospital with terminal lung cancer:

> *'I have been the recipient of an extraordinary array of human and humane responses to my plight. These acts of kindness – the simple human touch from my caregivers have made the unbearable bearable.'*

In many cases, it does not take much to make the unbearable bearable, and it is not rocket science, as these simple acts of kindness and caring are often just that, simple. Therein, however, lies the rub. If medicine was solely about compassion and kindness, then treatments, cures and lives saved would be things of the past. The role of the doctor would revert to times past and become more pastoral, akin to the famous painting 'The Doctor' by Luke Fildes, where we see the values of an ideal, caring physician alongside the inadequacies of medical treatment. Medicine is about the practical application of scientific knowledge and is best practised when the science is entwined with the person-patient, in a caring embrace. The wise doctor will see *Cum Scientia Caritas* as an amalgam of two ends of a spectrum and avoid too much divergence from the mean during the course of a career.

32

HIPPOCRATIC HOLIDAYS

2019

This is something else. Dappled light on turquoise water, leafy Caribbean vegetation, bobbing craft moored alongside the path from Princess Margaret Beach to Port Elizabeth, Bequia. Picture perfect.

Annie and I are on the trip of a lifetime, visiting great friends in the Caribbean. Ambling along the beach path, a Gallery sign attracts our attention, and we stumble into the Nautical Art Museum of Patrick 'Doc' Chevailler: his vivid wall-to-wall aquamarine undersea canvasses are immediately arresting, but wait a minute. There, out of the corner of my eye, is a familiar sight. A home from home mirage.

An examination couch, mercury sphygmomanometer and stethoscope lurk in a side room. The 'Doc's' consulting room is all white linen and polished wooden floors, with a view of the beach behind a large oak desk. I am fascinated and keen to explore this most eclectic of medical facilities, a world away from my homogenised NHS life. Pushing forward, I quietly put my head around the white-panelled door, and there in front of me is a tidy clinical room stuffed with similar medical paraphernalia to what I have accumulated in Botesdale. There is a small hospital on the island, staffed by one visiting doctor on rotation, but otherwise the only other source of help is the 'Doc.' There are scores of medical artists in the world, such as our local Cambridge transplant surgeon Sir Roy Yorke Calne, but this is my first experience of an artist's studio juxtaposed with medical consulting room. How do patients access the Doc's services, and how does he juggle painting with his medical practice? I want to talk to the 'Doc' about his medical life, as I am bursting with questions, but there is an aloofness which I suspect is borne out of the fact that he sees that we are unlikely to make a purchase. Never mind, the memory of this deeply personal Parisian consulting room, found on the edge of a Caribbean beach, sticks with me. Have I ever worked with such a sense of individual freedom and work–life balance; in such a state of supposedly relaxed and singular autonomy for patient and physician alike?

Well, I suppose the closest I got to working on my tod as a lone doctor was whilst on call in Botesdale, on a Sunday morning in the late 80s. At this time, we ran a Sunday surgery staffed entirely by the on-call doctor, who was responsible for appointment booking, telephone enquiries, consultations, dispensing of medicine and visits. I enjoyed the purity of the clinical responsibility of the individual GP divorced from the burgeoning medical workforce and bureaucracy. Provided I was not swamped and overwhelmed by my workload, these Sunday mornings could be strangely rewarding and enjoyable. However, this modus operandi was unsustainable in an advancing NHS, driven by IT, data, performance scrutiny, teamwork, and shifts, never mind the fact that these Sundays could at times be utterly exhausting.

So, despite a romantic notion of relaxed holism and individualism à la the 'Doc,' I knew in my heart of hearts that this was an impossible dream in today's NHS. Possible whilst living beach side in the Caribbean, and maybe the UK in 1919, but not in Botesdale, not now in 2019. The NHS appears to be pulled along by an utilitarian philosophy, where the individual, as patient and clinician, is being superseded by the perceived greater good. Lone, single-handed GPs are now no more, with even single GP practices being subsumed into ever larger Primary Care Networks: 'Big is Beautiful' organisations, with the possible denial of community-facing continuity of care. Two philosophical theories – Kantian respect for autonomy and utilitarianism – battling it out once again in medical thinking, this time in primary care provision. Kant appears to be winning in the Caribbean at the moment, but not in the NHS presently. Let us hope that we can achieve a balanced, centrist position in the 2020s.

Closer to home, in France, and another consideration comes to mind: patient wellbeing during hospital confinement. Annie and I are high in the French Alps on the Plateau d'Assy near Mont Blanc. Quirky, I know, but we were not sightseeing or skiing but making a pilgrimage to view the sanatoria that litter the plateau. Opened in the 1920s and 30s, these facilities were a major line of defence in the constant battle against the 'Captain of all these Men of Death,' Tuberculosis. Futuristic even today, with architectural designs embracing the necessities of good food, fresh air and sunlight, these hospitals are a testament to the value of wellbeing in health care.

Annie and I have seen such European establishments before, where health in its broadest sense is embraced in the function and form of hospital design. We still talk of the hospital near Lake Garda, Italy, with balconies arranged outside each room to allow all patients to make full use of the sun and fresh air – to allow their Vitamin D levels to rocket. On exiting the hospital, we could not help but notice the industrial-sized waste disposal skips overflowing with wine bottles! 'Cin-cin!' On first inspection, incarceration in this hospital looked fun, despite the potential for a bashed-up liver courtesy of the ready supply of local Bardolino and Lugano wine.

In today's NHS, in the drive for greater efficiency, corseted by financial constraint, we seem to have forgotten the notion of patient wellbeing in hospital design and function. There were exceptions to this, of course, such as the Devonshire Royal Hospital in Buxton, with its hydrotherapy pools, balconies for patients and wonderful dome dwarfing that of St Paul's. When Annie and I visited in 1995, the hospital was in full throttle, with a notably uplifting ambience that both staff and patients seemed to enjoy. Sadly, this wing of the NHS Manchester rheumatology department closed its doors in 2000 and is now owned by the University of Derby.

The last of the hydrotherapy units that dotted the country is now no more. Interestingly, when visiting the Hospital de Sant Pau in Barcelona, designed by Catalan Modernisme architect Lluis Domenech, down the road from Gaudi's La Sagrada Familia, we learnt that the inspiration for ward design, ventilation and lighting were drawn from the London teaching hospitals, including my own alma mater, The Middlesex Hospital. So, despite the fact that we appear to have been keeping up with the pace in the past, it is maybe the case that nowadays general patient wellbeing during hospital admission is considered unimportant, as length of stays have declined. The first goal now is to prevent admission in the first place, and then if there is no alternative, ensure that discharge occurs ASAP!

OK, enough of this pontificating on the NHS response to wellbeing. Let us take a trip to Asia – the East Coast of Thailand – and review my hands-on and deeply personal healing experience. Annie and I were visiting a Healing Centre at a beach-side hotel on the small isthmus of Rai Leh Beach. Arriving at the reception, we were greeted by a pretty local lady offering a variety of massages. Head and neck for Annie and foot for me. I didn't have long to wait in my reclining chair, as from a side room came a strong-looking woman with a boxer's shoulders and brickie's hands. We conversed in sign language as I discarded my sandals and she set to work on my right foot:

Slap, slap, slap, slap. Ouch, ouch, ouch, ouch. What the hell!

I looked down at my foot, where the veins were standing out like blue whipcord. The surrounding skin was scarlet, my exposed ankle joint shrieking with pain. Any varicose veins pummelled into near rupture by the onslaught. This was torture worthy of the Stasi.

The rough hands now applied warm oil, more dermabrasion, depilation, and deforestation than massage. Ouch. Soreness.

A warm towel and relief, for what turned out to be a respite from the main course to come.

A tool was produced that looked like a small, hard piece of cork applied to the end of a stiff wire. Where is this tool heading, and what is it going to do? Which orifice, which cavity, which appendage? The mind was boggling. Next thing, it was pushed up hard against the end of the bone in my big toe, and I mean hard. Each toe in turn in fact. Ouch, ouch, five times.

Could it get worse? Yes. The toe joints were then flexed, and the tool was rammed into each joint space for what seemed like an eternity. Is this legal? Is this certified? What healing philosophy is this derived from? Guantanamo? Ouch.

I learnt to respect joint cartilage, and I remember an orthopaedic surgeon informing me that in the early stages of osteoarthritis a joint's surface becomes pitted, like a kitchen floor losing floor tiles. As more and more 'cartilage tiles' are lost, the underlying bone is increasingly exposed and the arthritis worsens. This conversation with the surgeon played through my mind during this 'healing therapy,' as I was losing my kitchen tiles by the second here, and what made it worse is that this session with the carpet fitter was costing me.

Finally, my foot massage was finished and a warm towel applied. I rested my head back on the reclining chair, relaxed and drew breath. Relief. Then the dawning of a terrible and distressing reality; I have another foot. Ouch, ouch again.

After another half an hour of this caper, I came out of that treatment room with the gait of a giraffe imitating a stork. Not normally aware of my feet, they were now screaming 'What the hell have you put us through?' Somebody had taken a flamethrower to my skin and a corkscrew to my toes and metatarsals. I was tottering along like a foot-binded Geisha, superficial and deep pain radiating up from my feet to my shins. I flopped into the swimming pool, where I found Annie declaring that her massage was a vigorous and relaxing session with the lady on the front desk. 'A delight, worth every penny. I feel so much better,' she said, floating serenely in the pool. Oh great!

Annie was informed that as well as providing healing therapies to tourists, the centre was also set up to provide refuge and work for women who were victims of domestic abuse in Bangkok. Sadly, the healing centre is no more, as less than four months after our visit, a tectonic plate shifted in the Indian Ocean that resulted in the Boxing Day tsunami which devastated the small, low-lying and vulnerable isthmus. Right place, right time for our family to visit a paradise. I can only hope my masseur was not anywhere near the refuge on that fateful morning.

33

PARTNERSHIP

2019

They do say that a GP partnership is a marriage without the sex. Well, usually without the sex, as I have heard of the occasional colleague who has pushed the boundaries a little bit in this regard. This metaphor arises from the long-term nature of the partnership, sustained through thick and thin, until retirement or death intervene. A band of brothers and sisters, until death do us part!

So it seemed apposite to be reflecting on my experiences of GP partnership during a celebratory meal for Tim on his retirement with the five central figures in my working life: Annie and I, along with partners Rob and Tim and their wives, Sue and Anna. For over twenty years, we were all in this venture together, working in a small village general practice; six individuals welded together by a common bond and shared past. Among the array of emotions on display that night in the restaurant was a sense within us all that we had migrated through our working lives together as a more or less coherent group and, despite the odd glitch, should be proud of the fact that we could still speak, never mind enjoy each other's company!

Tim has already made his presence felt on these pages; however, more needs to be said about Rob.

Calm and strategic, strong on integrity and family, he was the natural foil to the youthful impulses of his junior partners. For years, as senior partner, Rob led the troops through a long period of relative stability, with patient care and staff contentment top of the list of practice priorities. Looking back, these were the golden years, when we were relatively free from government interference to pursue our own professional path, with good patient care the daily goal. Rob was central to these gilded days.

Now, this is no primer on general practice, no business 'how to' book uniquely found in airports; however, writing these pages has made me reflect on the different facets of my working life, with partnership central to this process. What were the elements that went into the fact that we could all celebrate twenty years of working together? Here is my homespun and brief attempt to try and elucidate what makes a sustainable GP partnership – the mystical NHS modus operandi within primary care, which has baffled NHS business leaders, politicians and the wider public for years.

Unbeknown to many, general practice partnerships operate as self-employed businesses, rather than as salaried practitioners to the NHS, as is the case with our hospital colleagues. This status carries with it a degree of autonomy, as well as managerial responsibility and commitment. It is this commitment that is one of the great strengths of the partnership system, whereas the aforementioned autonomy can lead to bloody mindedness, giving rise to exasperation within the

NHS corridors of managerial power. Herding cats comes to mind.

Whatever the pros or cons of a partnership system, there is no doubt that whether as a small or, as more recently, large entity, smooth function, efficiency and drive is more likely to occur with a cohesive rather than a dysfunctional grouping of partners. In our case, Rob, Tim and I achieved probably the most in our partnership when the three of us were operating as a small cohesive unit.

Why was this? Well, I would suggest that first of all we shared similar basic values around patient care, respect for our families and staff, money and leisure, thereby allowing us to manage the practice with a shared, consistent voice. Translating this voice into a shared enterprise embraced by everyone within the practice helped foster an atmosphere of inclusion and immersion in line with the practice's caring ethos. As a partnership, we also tried to ensure that we were scrupulously open and fair in dealing with each other, especially around workload, finance and holidays. Anything other than an equal cutting of the cake leads to strife.

Not to say that we did not have problems, including interpersonal issues along the way. Of course we did; however, whether we either metaphorically punched each other to a standstill, knew when to stay out of harm's way, or simply grew older and wiser, for some reason the emotional bond between us grew and flourished. Glitches will happen between individuals, and as it is important to be open, honest and not afraid to speak up, conflict resolution without bearing grudges is vital in a partnership. Putting differences aside and looking to the future is imperative.

Having a stable partnership is all very well, but personnel will always change with time, necessitating time spent on recruitment. Bringing the right people into a GP practice, especially a small one, is crucial, in that everyone has an important role to play. The wrong person can easily upset the apple cart and create more work and stress for everyone else. It is also important to understand the strengths and weaknesses of the team and bring in individuals whose attributes, skills and personality add to the mix. I frequently struggled with the fine detail of practice management and so rejoiced when this was done by someone else!

Finally, it is really important to down tools and retire at the opportune time, both for the individual but also for the practice. Not everyone has the luxury of being able to retire at a specific time, but if the option is available, then timing is important. Recently, in these times of paucity of workforce, I have seen practices with partners all of the same age retire in a matter of months, leaving one poor soul to carry the can. Ideally, there should be a few years between each retirement to allow for a new team to coalesce and develop. Conversely, I have also seen practices where a partner rumbles on for too long, stifling the development of the practice.

Sounds all too easy, doesn't it, when sketched out here. However, managing a general practice, with the responsibility partnership brings, can be onerous. I was very grateful in having competent and kind Rob and Tim around me for the majority of my working life, and I'm not sure I would have made it through without them. A retirement meal out was a small way of acknowledging and celebrating this unique relationship. As the six of us drift off into the foothills of our retirement, following differing experiences and byways, I know we will take time to come together, chew the cud, and share each other's spirit and stories, until death really does us part.

34

THE ONE AND ONLY ALBERT …

CONVERSATIONS WITH MY ALTER EGO
2020

'I am sorry, Dr Yager. I don't think it is possible to train Albert to walk to heel yet. He might benefit from more time on all aspects of dog training.'

More time? All aspects?

This was the tenth class, and we had got nowhere with our blue roan Cocker Spaniel. Even Linda, the instructor, had given up.

'OK, so what would you suggest, Linda?,' I queried.

'I think he needs another session of classes at least.'

'Another ten sessions?'

'Yes.'

That sounds expensive.

'Will that really help?'

Hope springs eternal.

'It won't do any harm, although I suspect you will have your work cut out. I am not sure Albert will ever really walk to heel,' replied Linda in a faltering tone.

Not exactly a ringing endorsement of the sessions. Do we cut and run? Is it Albert, or are we rubbish at this? I think it is a bit of both.

Let's cut and run.

Am I being a tight arse?

'Thanks Linda, we'll discuss it and get back to you.'

Linda and I knew, and maybe even Albert knew, we wouldn't be back.

A decision we came to regret!

'How is Albert?' enquired Carol one morning in the surgery.

'Yeah, he is fine thanks. As much of a scamp as ever.'

I don't like where this is heading. Try and keep calm.

'We love it when Albert comes round to see us. In fact, we have got some special treats for him ready and waiting! All sorts.'

Special treats. All sorts. What the hell is going on here, Carol!

'Do you mean Albert visits your house a lot?'

'Oh, yes quite a lot. We are always happy to see him though. We love him.'

You love him? This sounds as though quite a relationship has been struck up. Move on, Andrew, with the consultation, while I process this in the back of my mind.

Hang on a minute. Maybe Carol would keep him and adoption is a serious possibility. Must talk to Pom about this option.

Near neighbours Carol and John were lovely, gentle people. Albert had a habit of running off, despite multiple attempts to fence in the garden, but the routine nature of his visits shook me up a bit. This was not the first time I had been left short for words as far as Albert was concerned and would not be the last. More of the same coming up.

Early on a Saturday morning, the phone rings.

'Hello, do you have a dog called Albert?'

'Yes.'

'Good, this is Stowmarket vets here. We would be grateful if you could come and pick him up as soon as possible. Somebody found him and has brought him in,' said a woman in a stern, admonishing tone.

Silence from my end as I collected myself and cleared my throat.

Normally WE ring the vet. I hope this isn't a scam call? If not, we are in trouble.

'Thank you, we will be down immediately,' I replied, more than slightly subserviently.

Stowmarket! I don't believe this. Had he walked there?

Stowmarket was 12 miles away! Albert had escaped the previous night, and we had spent much of the night looking for him.

How do we explain this one away?

The short drive down seemed interminable.

'Which of us is going into to collect him, Pom?'

I really don't want to do this. I am strangely afraid of the vet. This seems like a borderline safeguarding issue. Have we been negligent?

'I'll do it, Andrew.'

Annie is always the strong, steadfast one. Phew.

'Thanks, Pom.'

Coward.

Shirley on the health centre reception desk phones me in my consultation room.

'Hello, Andrew, there is a policeman here in reception, with Albert in his car! Somebody reported him wandering around the village. The policeman has to get going. Can you come out and see to him please, now?'

Jesus, Albert.

First make an apology to the patient sitting in front of me.

Try and brush it off with the policeman as a one-off event.

Will I be accused of wasting police time?

Try and not worry the health centre staff. Pretend it is all sorted, even if we know it's not. He could be off again tonight!

I got Albert from the policeman at reception and quickly took him home.

Oh no, there is the patient still waiting in my consulting room patiently. Offer more apologies.

Must revisit the adoption idea with Pom.

Try to concentrate, Andrew.

'Hello, Andrew, this is Ted here. We have got Albert with us. Can you come and pick him up, please. No rush, as he has shared my breakfast of bacon and eggs. I am due to go out soon, but he can come in the car with me if you can't make it for a while.'

God, Ted is a nice guy, but bacon and eggs is a bit extreme. Show gratitude, Andrew, keep quiet about the bacon and eggs, and yes to the trip for Albert in the car. Anything to keep him busy.

'Hello, is that the owner of a little dog called Albert. We have him here in the churchyard, and we can hold him here until you come and get him.'

There are so many really nice people in this village.
Thank you.

Were they the same people who showed up at the door with Albert last month? Must check with Pom and run the adoption issue past her again.

Exasperated neighbour: 'Hello, I have brought Albert back. He has just eaten our cat's food . . . again!'

The only way out of this, Andrew, is to keep offering profuse apologies and say we hope it won't happen again. I know, they know that is not true. Offer to replace the cat food? Try and look sincere about this. Am I smirking?

Exasperated daughter: 'Dad, Albert has just eaten my giant Easter Egg . . . again!'

I know, I know, chocolate is bad for dogs, but Albert would always seem to find the stuff hidden in the children's bedrooms and thrived on it.

Keep my head down on this one. It's the only way to avoid yet another family conflagration. Chocolate is bad for dogs, but Albert appears immune. Why?

Nine-year-old Albert bursts into the dining room as I'm trying to catch a nesting jackdaw that has fallen down our chimney. Now, though Albert was more show than working Cocker, did he in any way show interest in the bird careering around the room? Did he join the chase?

No, is the short answer. What, then, did he do in his bid to help the situation? Well, he promptly squatted down and crapped not once but twice in quick succession on the floor and then cocked his leg on the door frame before trotting out.

Oh no, there are bird feathers mixed in with dog shit. I can't even begin to think of catching the bird without clearing up the mess first. This floor is a warzone. Where is the kitchen roll and the Flash? Where is the jackdaw now?

What the hell, Albert?

Time to offer some much-needed mitigation. Albert was not our first experience of dog ownership. On this note, our other dog, Labrador Paddy, came top of the ten-session aforementioned training class.

OK, we were not obsessional about it, but we hoped to offer them a loving family home. It is just that Albert was driven by an overwhelming olfactory sense that blinded him to higher brain function: in his own forceful way, he was unique, a force of nature, more suited to a sniffer dog than domestic pet. It seemed that his wanderings resulted more from the pull of random smells, maybe kilometres away, than any desire to run off or escape, a function of the 200-plus million olfactory receptor cells (50 times that of a human), as well as an extra smell organ, the vomeronasal organ, situated just above the mouth.

You are kidding. Do you seriously believe this brief explanation helped your exasperation and anxiety, Andrew?

No, not at all, actually.

Annie and I always greeted Albert's return with a sense of relief and deep gratitude. In these days of perceived dog abuse and theft, we were struck by the general kindness and civility shown towards Albert by our fellow citizens. Maybe it's an oxytocin thing, but the relationship between canines and humans is truly remarkable.

Humankind is not that bad after all. Albert had become a village favourite. The British love their dogs.

Maybe I was getting used to this situation.

The generosity and patience shown by a multitude of neighbours and patients who took the time to help Albert was always appreciated, if tinged with a touch of embarrassment.

I should have stopped worrying what the patients thought, which was probably 'Old Dr Yager is crap at looking after Albert. He can't even keep him in the garden. I think he is better with us lot.'

This would all have been so much easier if I didn't live in the village. There again, the patients were always really forgiving about this. God bless them.

Sadly, Albert suffered a leaking mitral valve, common to Cocker Spaniels in old age, and despite treatment, he died recently of heart failure. Courageous, cheerful and positive to the very end, he is missed by our family, as well as half of the village of Rickinghall. Annie considers getting Albert safely to old age as having been more stressful than raising all our three children put together and is thus one of her greatest life achievements.

Despite everything, Albert, we miss you, and adoption was never seriously on the cards. You were a remarkably positive and spirited little dog. Listen to St Peter, don't stray too far from those Pearly Gates, and rest in peace.

35

BARRY

2021

My final story started over three decades ago and is still unfolding now. Annie and I reminisced on this when attending a 30-year memorial service for Barry, surrounded by a remarkable family and group of friends. Casting my mind back, I remember Barry as a force of nature. A vibrant, confident property developer in his mid-thirties, striding into my consulting room and complaining of tingling in his hand. Sadly, within days, his condition deteriorated, requiring admission to hospital. A diagnosis of a brain tumour was made, requiring surgery, radiotherapy and chemotherapy.

On discharge from hospital, I went round to visit Barry and found him sitting in a small snug alongside wife Nuala, small children Dominic and Holly, and an attentive group of friends. Despite the desperate nature of the situation, I was struck by Barry's determination to fight his condition, and the support he was receiving in his resolve from everyone around him. I have never seen anything quite like the way this group of friends provided support to the family, either before or since. They were prepared to drop everything and give time, energy and love to Barry, Nuala and the children. Total commitment, with a happy resolve. Despite the tragic circumstances surrounding my visits to this family, entering the house was like sinking into a warm pool of human kindness and goodwill, engendered by this special family and friendship group. I would leave the house feeling sad but strangely uplifted by what I had just witnessed; human friendship at its best. Of course, this aura was no accident, with Barry and Nuala placing an absolute value on family bonds and friendship, alongside a remarkable ability to bring people together and foster good relationships. The more visits I undertook, the more I was being drawn into this circle of friendship, this pool of human warmth, which little did I realise would last a lifetime.

Barry battled on with a smile and a calmness that belied his desperate circumstances, again supported by Nuala, close friends and our excellent district nurses and night sitters. There was no doubt, however, that Barry's condition was slowly deteriorating, day by day, with decisions needing to be made by Barry and Nuala around end of life, resuscitation and place of care. There is a strong governmental drive for patients to have the choice of dying at home, with target levels to match. Not everyone wants to stay at home, though, and if social and family support is unavailable, looking after someone in their own home in their final days and weeks can be emotionally and physically challenging for all concerned. There is a widely held perception that the community palliative care services will provide such support; however, in many areas of the country, unless there is good back up from friends and family, remaining at home can be problematic, and on many occasions impossible. Each case has to be judged individually as to whether the patient remains at home or goes into care, according to the patient's wishes, clinical situation and access to support. There is no right or wrong, with arbitrary targets meaningless to those individuals dealing with end of life care day by day on the ground. As far as Barry was concerned, he wanted to stay as close to his family as possible for every minute of every day, so this meant staying at home. Nuala wanted Barry by her side and had the fortitude and resolve to look after him and the children. Our small medical and nursing team were able to provide clinical support, whilst the other family members and friends provided ongoing practical and emotional support. If end of life care at home failed under these circumstances, then there was no hope for the rest of us!

In Barry's final days, I was visiting once or twice a day, and on a cold winter's lunchtime, I intimated to Nuala that he had only hours to live and resolved to return at the end of my evening surgery. On arrival later on, Barry's life force was nearly spent, and there by his bedside was Nuala offering calming words and loving comfort whilst he slowly made his final journey and peacefully stopped breathing. A hushed calm spread over the house as we all reflected on Barry, his life and death. Then Nuala and a few friends spoke up and said that Barry had discussed this moment many times and wanted everyone to have a drink and toast his life, rather than drown in grief. This expression of life, love and joy felt totally appropriate, with a group of us celebrating a life well lived in a welter of love and emotion. Again, I was struck by the fact that dying in hospital would have made this spontaneous expression difficult, and it was further vindication of the decision to keep Barry at home, where he had been looked after through thick and thin. After a while, I took my leave with a few final words regarding undertakers and death certificates. Venturing out into the cold evening air, I realised all too late when my legs buckled that I had had too much alcohol in a relatively short space of time. I fortunately returned home safe and sound. Annie was taken aback by the slightly inebriated and flushed figure in the kitchen, fresh from a palliative care visit!

Eventually, Nuala, Dominic and Holly moved away and slowly worked through their grief with the help of their ever-present family and friends, assisted several years later by Ray, who joined the family as Nuala's wonderful husband. How do I know all of this? Well don't forget that I had been immersed into the warmth of Nuala's friendship group whilst looking after Barry, and, more to the point, with time so was Annie. When meeting up with Nuala, Barry and the past were never far from our thoughts; however, our friendship was strongly based in the present and future, with new ventures to share. As I have intimated before, once you are in Nuala's friendship group, you are well and truly in. And so, we have been to parties, wedding celebrations and more recently Barry's 30-year memorial service, mentioned at the start of this tale. As a group, we have all got older and moved on, with life changing immeasurably in so many ways. Except that in some ways life hasn't changed. Humans come together, form relationships, and sadly at times depart from each other: the poignancy of this human flow is not lost on me, especially when attending a service in memory of Barry surrounded by familiar faces.

36

POSTSCRIPT

2021

I am sat at my desk with the glazed eyes, sweaty sheen and hunched back of the serial Zoomer and serial Teamer. Another day, another long list of meetings slumped over my computer working for the CCG and Macmillan on cancer pathways. The new normal of the remote worker post Covid pandemic. Better this, however, than the poor devils who, with Covid 19 lurking around every corner, head out daily into harm's way to keep our society on the rails. Covid has arrived and transformed our world to devastating effect: individuals, families, businesses and governments. Few areas have escaped viral scrutiny, with any societal dysfunction pre-pandemic highlighted and punished.

Our society has experienced profound disruption, disturbance and transformation, with general practice not escaping covid's metaphorical cosh. As such, many of the stories told in this collection not only arise from previous decades, but from a more immersive, interactive and personal but less fraught and frantic time. A viral and virtual sledgehammer has been taken to much of what I have written about so far. My thirty-year journey has gone from pen and ink, phone boxes and lone working at night, to a digital, data-driven, interconnected world with remote working and hotly disputed virtual transactional appointments. Coupled with this is the relinquishing by the profession in 2004 of the 24-hour commitment of general practice to each individual patient, which has led to the erosion of the vocational and relational foundation on which late twentieth-century general practice was built. Despite personally benefiting from the 2004 contract, as long nights and weekends on call were now a thing of the past for me, I can see that many of the values underpinning general practice have changed. Sadly, these twin upsets of cultural change and Covid have made many areas of our society question the role of general practice. I fear that the general practice that I witnessed is now on thin ice. Yet the central tenets of general practice are the same, in that the system delivers a patient in front of a generalist, where communication skills, clinical expertise, continuity of care and considered conscientiousness are paramount. Surely it is not too late to discover a modern modus operandi. For sure, AI, remote working, allied health professionals and practice teams will all play a part; however, for me there are three changes that need to happen to revive UK general practice. Firstly, funding (not salaries) needs to be increased to allow for consultation times to be at least 15 minutes, in line with other Western countries. GP numbers and funding need to be based around this formula for change. Secondly, the powers that be within general practice, such as the RCGP and BMA, need to rediscover and generate a societal contract with the patient and embrace continuous care to the individual patient. Finally, if this vocational, relational status is enhanced then central government needs to respect this re-evaluated professional position and allow general practice to function more autonomously.

So, there we have it. A collection of vignettes illustrating the thoughts and career path of a slightly eccentric and accident-prone GP who just happened to wash up in lovely Suffolk. On the whole, I have enjoyed my general practice career, as it has undoubtedly been rewarding and allowed me to look after my family, but the time has come to look forward, finish reminiscing and truly embrace the future.

As Annie and I move on, we remain children of the NHS and proud of our combined eighty years of service.

November 2021

Thank you to all of my family, friends and colleagues who have helped and contributed to these stories with enormous patience and care. A special thank you also to the people of North Suffolk, who welcomed Annie and I into their midst all of those years ago.

Printed in Great Britain
by Amazon

21796841R00128